AROUND THE
CIRCLE
One More Time

A journey living through mental illness, abuse, and the power of forgiveness and hope

Darlene Hansen

Inscript

Inscript Books
A Division of Dove Christian Publishers
PO Box 611
Bladensburg, MD 20710-0611

Dove Christian Publishers
Attn: Permissions
P.O. Box 611
Bladensburg, MD 20710-0611
www.dovechristianpublishers.com

Paperback ISBN 978-1-957497-56-3

Inscript and the portrayal of a pen with script are trademarks
of Dove Christian Publishers.

Printed in the United States of America

This is a work of nonfiction. The events are portrayed to
the best of the author's memory. While all the stories in
this book are true, some names and identifying details
have been changed to protect the privacy of the people involved.

I dedicate this book to Larry,
with gratitude and appreciation
for your willingness and determination to grow.
Thank you for the courage and support
you've given for me to share our story.
I am honored to celebrate life with you.
To our amazing children,
thank you for the consistent love,
honor and respect you've given to us
as your parents throughout your lives.
My prayer is for each of your homes to be blessed
and your marriages to always be filled with
Faith, Hope, and Love.

Contents

Foreword vii

Chapter 1
Midlife Crisis 1

Chapter 2
The Journey Begins 4

Chapter 3
Never Forgotten 8

Chapter 4
The Sin of Presumption 11

Chapter 5
Marital Bliss 14

Chapter 6
The Honeymoon is Over 17

Chapter 7
Where the Rubber Meets the Road 22

Chapter 8
A Bridge Over Troubled Waters 29

Chapter 9
So Quickly Forgotten 36

Chapter 10
Heading West 40

Chapter 11
The Last Place on Earth 45

Chapter 12
On the Road Again 51

Chapter 13
Heading South 60

Chapter 14
Resurrection From the Rubble 67

Chapter 15
Heading Further South 76

Chapter 16
A New Foundation..81

Chapter 17
Jerusalem, Judea and Samaria.....................86

Chapter 18
Flipped and Toppled.......................................92

Chapter 19
The Uttermost Parts of the Earth.............102

Chapter 20
North, South, East, or West?....................107

Chapter 21
 A Mission in My Backyard........................116

Chapter 22
The Grass Withers, the Flower Fades.....122

Chapter 23
Expanding our Territory.............................127

Chapter 24
A Time for Miracles.....................................132

Chapter 25
Time to Build..141

Chapter 26
Another Time Around?................................147

Chapter 27
 Days to Cherish..153

Chapter 28
More Than Imagined...................................159

Chapter 29
Waiting On the Wind....................................163

Chapter 30
The Path Ahead...167

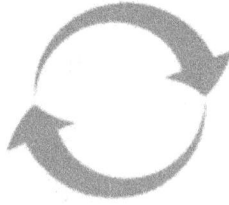

FOREWORD

Proverbs 4:18 promises, "But the path of the righteous is like the light of dawn that shines brighter and brighter until the full day."[1]

Life is a journey.

In planning a road trip, I am the type of person who gathers information and maps out the entire route ahead of time. I try to eliminate all possible obstacles and control all variables to stay safe. I detail events in advance to know when to start and stop and allow sufficient time for meals and activities. I want to have an enjoyable trip by avoiding detours and roadblocks and staying far away from avalanches. I love an organized and predictable life.

I believe most people seek a lifelong partner who shares the same values and agrees to work together toward an ultimate destination from point A to point B. I am no exception. However, no one can plan ahead for mental illness. On the day I declared my wedding vows, I could never have anticipated my future ahead. Mine is an extremely impulsive co-pilot who rarely plans and changes his mind frequently. This makes traveling together quite tricky. There have been times when I felt as if the steering wheel of our life's travel

---

1   Unless otherwise identified, all Scripture quotations in this publication are taken from the HOLY BIBLE, NEW AMERICAN STANDARD version Copyright c 1960,1962,1963, 1968, 1971, 1972, 1973, 1975, 1977, 1995 by THE LOCKMAN FOUNDATION A corporation not for profit, La Habra. CA, All Rights Reserved

vehicle was unexpectedly hijacked, sending us into a crazy tailspin.

Roundabouts are designed to keep the flow of traffic going and prevent delays in intersections, but if the driver does not know how to exit the maze, the duration of the trip can be extended by going around in circles, heading out in the wrong direction, or even causing an accident through confusion. This can make the trip extremely frustrating and dangerous.

Other than the regular family arguments, I did not experience any domestic violence in my childhood home environment. When it became my reality after marriage, it caught me off guard. As a youngster growing up in the Church, I believed that most adults who attended weekly had their acts together, like the "Leave it to Beaver" model. However, as an adult, I have become aware that verbal and physical abuse in the Christian home is more commonplace than I had ever imagined and is rarely talked about in Christian circles.

The subject matter is often taboo, and as a result, countless people suffer in silence, believing that no one can relate to or understand them.

It says in James 5:16, **"Confess your sins to one another, and pray for one another so that you may be healed. The effective prayer of a righteous man (or woman) can accomplish much."** But when the hurt remains in the dark, no healing occurs. Although it has taken me many years, I have, at last, learned that God created us to live in community, to share our trials and victories, and to support and pray for one another.

God loves us so much and wants us to live out our lives to the fullest, experiencing freedom and all His good plans and purposes. That is why the devil fights so hard to keep us isolated and hiding our hurts in the darkness. If he cannot rob us of our salvation, he will do all he can to take away our joy, peace, and effectiveness in God's kingdom. John 10:10 says, **"The thief comes only to steal and kill and destroy; I came so that they would have life and have it abundantly."**[1]

It took me many years to get up the courage to write this book. Shame prevented me from sharing the details of my earlier life. This delayed my own healing, along with that of my family. It robbed me of the fellowship that God desired me to enjoy with others. When I finally gained the valor to share my testimony and bring the truth into the light, I became aware of so many lies that had kept me bound for decades. I have not trained for, nor do I have, a mental health degree. I do, however, have lots of life experiences to share.

I have walked through years of pain and made many mistakes, but the good news is that healing and restoration are on the horizon for all of us who persevere.

I invite you to join me on my life journey. My hope and prayers are that, in some way, sharing my experiences can shed light on your path, help eliminate possible roadblocks, and illuminate the way for you to walk in new freedom.

Be blessed,

Darlene

A Message from my Husband

I would like to add this preface:

As you will witness in the pages ahead, Darlene and I have experienced years of hurt, accusation, bitterness, and unforgiveness. We've received much healing but have not yet arrived at perfection. God has brought us through these trials to use them for His glory. We are still learning by God's grace.

I share Darlene's vision for our story to be used for others to learn. I give my blessing for my wife to share her story, and I pray along with her for God to use this book as a tool for change in the lives of those He leads to read it.

Sincerely,

Larry

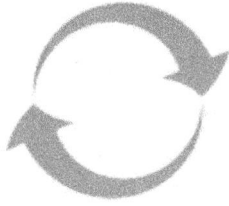

Chapter 1

MIDLIFE CRISIS

Yeah, I know this is a strange way to start a book, but my story begins in a place of confusion, internal conflict, and misery.

I was in a far-off country, anticipating a new chapter in my life. It was to be a season of answered prayers and long-awaited payoffs for deferred hopes and dreams, but it didn't quite pan out the way I had expected. This crisis was nothing I could've ever planned for or imagined.

> *October 29, 2005, journal entry: "This is SO hard. Everything inside me says, 'Deny yourself.' I know Your Word says that too. I have always tried to live according to Your Word. That's why this painful conflict is inside me. I do want to be free. I know You want me to be free. It can only happen with Your supernatural revelation. I trust You. It hurts. My head hurts, my heart hurts. My insides hurt. I need to start over. Show me the place. Hold me. I'm broken. I'm being ripped apart."*

I wrote these words in Ituziangó, a district of Buenos Aires, Argentina. My husband, Larry and I were about six weeks into a Youth With A Mission (YWAM) Discipleship Training School.

I had celebrated my forty-fifth birthday the previous month, and Larry had just turned fifty-three. We'd both resigned from our jobs in Mesa, Arizona, a couple of months earlier and traveled to the Southern Hemisphere, where we hoped to obtain training and seek God for our future.

I considered myself spiritually mature and was looking forward to new, insightful, and deeper teachings. I was especially expectant for my husband—who, in my opinion, had loads to learn both in his spiritual life and interpersonal relationships. That being the case, I was shocked when our training lessons were so basic. I couldn't imagine why a mission school filled with more than forty-five Christian students would need to teach a class entitled, "You Must Be Born Again"?

That was so very elementary! The instructor even used an object lesson that I considered quite childish: a railway train complete with an engine, coal car, and caboose, meant to symbolize how our life can be led or propelled.

The idea being taught was that each person has a body, soul, and spirit. We can be led by our flesh (intellect and desires), our soul (will and emotions), or our spirit (new creation). Moving the train cars around, the instructor explained how our flesh can be an enemy of our spirit. "When we are born again," he told us, "our flesh does not automatically submit to the Spirit of God. It's a matter of one's own free will. Filtering decisions through the flesh or intellect can prevent an individual from walking in obedience and following the Spirit of God, because the things of the Spirit are foolishness to the natural man, as explained in 1 Corinthians 2:14."

I knew that fleshly desires could lead to sin, but I never thought that researching, planning, and offering suggestions to others could be sinful. I knew that it made me angry when I felt controlled, but I had never considered myself to have a controlling personality. After all, I had never tried to put pressure on others. Wasn't my true intent to help my family and other people make "good choices"? So, for all

2

these years, had I really been walking by the Spirit, or was I actually walking in the flesh?

Suddenly, I found myself in a messy, painful dilemma. I cried for days, doubled up in a fetal position in my bed, faced with the truth of the ugliness inside of me. I was full of pride and years of beliefs that had left me confused.

Had my life been a total waste? After years of what I had thought to be faithfulness, how did I come to this crisis?

"As the deer pants for the water brooks,
So my soul pants for You, O God.
My soul thirsts for God, for the living God;
When shall I come and appear before God?
My tears have been my food day and night,
While they say to me all day long,
'Where is your God'?"
Psalms 42:1-3

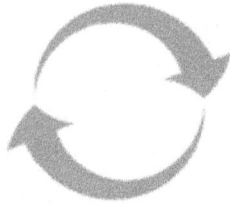

Chapter 2

THE JOURNEY BEGINS

I always knew that God loved me.

I was one of the fortunate ones who was born into a Christian family. From my earliest memories, I was in church. We attended both Sunday mornings and nights and also participated in Wednesday evening services. I was on the "Cradle Roll" as an infant and toddler and later graduated to Sunday School, where I was taught by flannelgraph all the Bible stories from Creation to Revelations.

My parents reinforced a healthy, Christian upbringing at home by implementing family devotions and bedtime prayers. This wasn't without impact. I remember one night around my sixth birthday, I acknowledged my sinful heart and asked Jesus to forgive me and become my personal Savior.

Our church was very mission-minded, and our family frequently entertained visiting missionaries for meals. At times, we even invited them to spend the night with us. I was glued to their exciting stories of adventure and evangelism and was convinced that there could be nothing more fulfilling than being a missionary. Therefore, I pledged my heart as a child, saying, "Here am I; send me!"

As far back as I can remember, my mom and dad modeled the example of sharing our talents. We were taught that each of us had been given abilities to develop and to bless others with them. We were given a small amount of allowance each week for doing our weekly chores and were encouraged to give the first part back to God, saving a portion for ourselves while always being willing to share with others in need. The idea of stewardship carried over into discovering our interests and natural abilities.

From a young age, I began singing with my dad and taking piano lessons with the intention of using them in ministry. We were also encouraged to help our neighbors and, indeed, anyone who needed assistance. Also, my parents demonstrated the gift of hospitality by hosting meals at our home nearly every weekend. The foundation laid down for my life's path was based on truth and love. This led to a sense of security and purpose and produced fond memories.

My Dad had a great and witty, although sarcastic, sense of humor. His favorite cartoon was the Road Runner Show, and each time the coyote would wipe out, Dad would laugh and laugh until tears ran down his face. I would join in on the fun but not quite understand why it was all so hilarious, since the tragedy could always be easily anticipated. I stood in awe at the way my dad was so quick to respond with funny comments, both with our family and out in public. We did have a good time together back in those days, and due to my father's early influence, I also inherited a very sarcastic sense of humor.

Since I was the eldest of four children, I was given the responsibility of keeping an eye on my two younger brothers and little sister. At that time, we were living in the healthy, rural countryside of Elmira, Oregon. We were free to run, scream, and build forts on our 9-acre property. There were frogs and water dogs to find in our natural springs, and we could play outside without fear until dusk. We knew all our neighbors and had no need to lock our doors. How could life be any better?

Then, shortly before entering junior high, my dad's job transferred him to the big city of Portland. So that we'd remain within our element of fir trees, my parents decided to settle in the beautiful and prestigious community of Lake Oswego, Oregon. There couldn't have been a place more culturally shocking anywhere on the face of the earth!

Dad was busy with his new supervisory position and was rarely home. My mom became involved in numerous activities in our brand-new church. I didn't fit into the unfamiliar environment well, but soon discovered through my "liberal" and "enlightened" teachers that I was simply a product of my environment. It was natural for me to believe the things I was taught growing up, but what was good for my parents and grandparents, they asserted, may not be good for me. This sounded reasonable, and I bought the lie hook, line, and sinker.

I remember reading a book at age fourteen that I had no business reading. I felt conviction, but then quickly excused myself, believing that it was because of my upbringing. I dismissed my uncomfortable conscience and continued the book, never to be bothered again by the uneasiness. In fact, I had decided at that point that there must not really be a god after all. I needed to find out—for Darlene's sake—what I believed and what made me happy. This led me to lie quite often to my parents, but that was alright; after all, I was setting out to try all that life had to offer me.

I graduated from High School in 1978 and quickly moved out with a friend to share an apartment. I attended community college with the plan of becoming an international flight attendant and traveling the world.

THE JOURNEY BEGINS

"Incline your ear and hear the words of the wise,
And apply your mind to my knowledge;
For it will be pleasant
if you keep them within you,
That that they may be ready on your lips.
So that your trust may be in the Lord,
I have taught you today, even you."
Proverbs 22:17-19

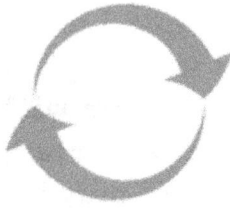

Chapter 3

NEVER FORGOTTEN

So, for nearly five years, I truly didn't hear the voice of God, nor did I see His hand in my life or the lives of others. In high school, I studied Spanish and French, hoping that one day I would use them during international travel, but I had completely forgotten about my childhood commitment to be used by my Creator.

After moving into my apartment, the thought never entered my mind to attend church. I worked, partied, and lived a life totally disparate from that of my upbringing. I continued to pursue my conversational Spanish in college, with plans to live and travel in South America.

It's worth mentioning here that through it all, I had the most amazing grandmother, who may not have known the details of my life but, nonetheless, never ceased to pray for me—together with all her other grandchildren and friends far and wide. I'm sure her prayers, along with those of others, led to the miracle of God speaking and my hearing.

One day, in September 1979, the week prior to my 19th birthday, while watching the evening news on T.V., I found myself listening to a report of possible war pending and hostages being held in Iran. My thoughts flashed back to some teachings of my early childhood. I clearly heard God say, "I'm real. What you were taught is accurate. The Bible is true. I'm coming back soon. You need to decide for your-self." When I heard this, I knew that I knew. I can't explain what or how it happened, but it was a miracle. I repented and was instantly transformed.

My former roommate probably wonders to this day what happened to me. My music, activities, and speech all changed in a moment. I set out to find a church and immediately remembered my pledge as a youngster, asking God to send me. Once again, I dared to believe that He could use me. I began researching Bible schools that offered training to evangelize children, hoping to use my Spanish overseas as a missionary.

Shortly after this encounter with God, I attended a singles get-together for Thanksgiving. During the conversation, I mentioned I was looking for a church home. A young man named Larry was there; he informed me that he'd been at-tending a church in my hometown and invited me to go with him. I agreed, and he arranged to pick me up the following weekend.

Upon meeting as planned, I was uncomfortable and totally freaked out as Larry gifted me with a rose and gold cross necklace. It was apparent that his intentions were more than being church mates, and we definitely weren't on the same wavelength! I did like the church, however, and soon became part of a young adults' group there but decided to take my own car. Larry saw me occasionally at church and invited me to do things with him, but I declined.

Before the end of the year, I had applied to a school in Warrenton, MO. I was accepted to attend The Child Evan-gelism Fellowship Leadership Training Institute to begin the following year in February 1980.

The devil attempted to disrupt my plans by sending a charming, wealthy man my way who talked the talk but didn't walk the walk. He asked me to marry him shortly after meeting at church, and I fell into the trap. Still, I wanted to keep my commitment to attending the mission school amidst my fiancé's protests. He was able to convince me, however, to move my personal items into his home prior to my leaving, reasoning that we had already set our wedding date shortly after my graduation and return home.

During this six-month time apart, I had the opportunity to grow in grace, knowledge, and wisdom. I also received spiritual counsel, which gave me the courage to call off the marriage engagement. While I was away at school, Larry had taken it upon himself to meet my parents and family and had also begun to attend their church.

I graduated with honors from CEF with plans to continue pursuing mission work with children. After returning home, it was made clear to my intended that my plans had changed, and I wouldn't be marrying him.

This meant moving all my personal belongings from my former boyfriend's home, which was a terrifying experience. I was offered the opportunity to move back in with my parents during this transition. My father was such a support to me, helping with the move and protecting me from abuse and accusations. He even helped me to obtain a much-needed legal restraining order. During this time, Larry continued to build relationships with my family, tried to be a friend and offer emotional support during the break-up, and actually started coming across a little less "freaky."

I finally felt like I had cleared the detour and was stepping back on track, facing a bright, exciting, and hopeful future!

**"The plans of the heart belong to man,
But the answer of the tongue is from the Lord.
All the ways of a man are clean in his own sight,
But the Lord weighs the motives.
Commit your works to the Lord,
And your plans will be established."
Proverbs 16:1-3**

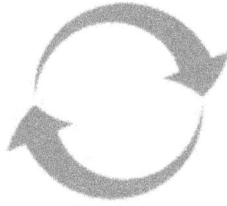

Chapter 4

THE SIN OF PRESUMPTION

After settling back into my parents' home, I began praying for direction. I was invited to teach a weekly children's Bible club in a nearby town. I was delighted with the experience and opportunity, and since it was a big undertaking, I was thankful that my friend Larry was willing to take the afternoons off from work and drive the distance to help each week. Our friendship kept growing, and although I made it clear that I wasn't interested in more than friendship, I guess Larry didn't believe me, because it wasn't long before he asked me to marry him. I declined.

It seemed he'd respected my answer, as he was still willing to help with the Bible club. Concluding our times together, he'd suggest reading the Bible together. I agreed to it, and each time we ended with prayer. Larry didn't take "no" for an answer, however. During one of these devotional times, he asked me again for a second time to marry him. I again blatantly denied his request.

As weeks went by, I started to feel more pressure from Larry. I explained my vision numerous times for overseas mission work, but Larry responded that Jesus gave us instruction to first be witnesses in Jerusalem, then Judea, Samaria, and then to the uttermost parts of the Earth. He argued that if we can't first be a witness in our own Jerusalem, then it may not be time to plan for going to the rest of the Earth. It did seem like he had a point there.

When I was growing up in the sticks of Elmira, I knew I was a little rough around the edges, but finishing my schooling in Lake Oswego had 'refined' me a bit and taught me some social etiquette. Larry, on the other hand, lacked social skills. He ate with his elbows on the table and chewed with his mouth open—while talking. He spoke over the top of friends in conversations and didn't pick up on any clues from people's body language. He'd get into others' personal space and would continue talking, even as he followed them away at times. I knew it was becoming necessary for me to take a stand about my feelings with Larry. He was kind and very helpful and I really did appreciate his giving heart. He was good with kids and very respectful to the elderly or handicapped. He was a very generous man, but on the other hand, seemed to have a very controlling personality. I didn't feel like my opinions were often respected. So, I needed to totally cut him off or decide if I should encourage him by continuing our friendship. Even though he was willing and diligent to help with Bible club, I often felt annoyed with him.

It was September, and I had just celebrated my 20th birthday. One evening, my mother came into my bedroom and asked a very strange question... This is how it kind of went:

<u>Mom</u>: Darlene, do you think you could learn to love Larry?
<u>Me:</u> Learn to love? That's an interesting question! (Thinking in my head ... hmmm ... God says we should even love our enemies!)
<u>Mom:</u> Maybe you could pray about it.
<u>Me:</u> OK. I'll pray.

In the days that followed, I thought about my conversation with my mom. Larry and I both grew up in the same church denomination and came from similar backgrounds.

We'd even attended the same church camp as kids. We had complementary values... But did we share the same vision for the future? I clearly remember the night I was on my knees in the dark living room, praying. (I don't often pray on my knees!) I tossed out this question to God, not expecting an answer: "God, do you want me to marry Larry?" I immediately heard the answer, "YES!"

Wow! That threw me for a loop! So, I began reasoning in my head... if God called me to be a missionary, and he wants me to marry Larry, He must be calling him to be a world missionary, too!

So, the presumption began.

"Who can discern his errors?
Acquit me of hidden faults.
Also keep back Your servant
from presumptuous sins;
Let them not rule over me;
Then I will be blameless,
And I shall be acquitted of great transgression."
Psalm 19:12-13

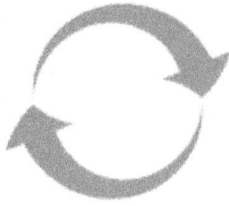

Chapter 5

MARITAL BLISS

Larry was so sure of himself that in October, he bought a wedding ring and had his personal diamond set in it. Next, he met with my dad and asked for my hand in marriage. He'd spent a lot of time with my parents, and my dad knew him pretty well. Dad gave his words of caution, wisdom, and counsel, but in the end, he gave his fatherly blessing. Having received the go-ahead, Larry arranged to pick me up from work to celebrate his 28th birthday on Oct 10th.

As soon as I got into the car, he excitedly popped the question while handing me the ring. I wasn't entirely surprised, and since God had already given me the OK, I answered this time in the affirmative. We initially decided on a March wedding. Spring would be nice and give us five months to prepare.

Upon hearing the news, my mother was delighted; however, her advice was, "If you're going to get married anyways, why not make it a December wedding and get a tax write-off?" So, December 6th, 1980, it would be. I was barely 20 years old.

Since there was a lot to do in less than two months, we resigned from our children's Bible Club. I got going right away on sewing my three bridesmaid dresses, as well as fabricating my own wedding gown and veil. I planned my dream wedding, which included singing a personal song to my groom and inserting the fruit of the Spirit into our holy wedding vows. Although I couldn't see it, I felt certain that God had many wonderful surprises awaiting me in marriage, including molding my future husband into all I had hoped for and dreamed of as a little girl. Of course, it was an unspoken fact that we would surely be united in heart and vision for ministry.

I knew Larry well enough to see he could become easily frustrated. I also understood—though not fully—that he struggled with some mental health challenges. Since that was out of my ballpark and God had told me to marry him, I believed God had some type of special plan to heal him and alleviate all of my annoyances.

In retrospect, I believed our marriage was more like an arranged one, not dependent upon the typical attractions experienced in the courting relationships of the West. But then, didn't the arranged marriages of the East have a higher survival rate, anyway? Like most women, I had high hopes for a "Happily Ever After" life.

Larry worked for his parents in the family jewelry business; December was the busy time of the year, so we were only allowed to plan a three-day weekend for our honeymoon, but we did have a nice celebration at the beach. Immediately after that, I moved promptly into Larry's house in the quiet, bedrock town of Canby, Oregon, to begin married life.

Having grown up hearing that feminists were evil and that a submissive wife is a virtuous wife, I tried to apply what I had learned. After marriage, I decided to change my legal name and signed my new checks as Mrs. Lawrence D. Hansen. In addition, I adopted an unhealthy notion that being in submission meant forgoing all of my personal interests and desires while giving in to every whim and fancy of my husband.

It didn't take me long to discover that my spending and saving habits were not on the same page as Larry's. I had a little nest egg saved up before our wedding, but after combining our assets and debts, I discovered Larry had three credit cards that he'd been carrying balances on monthly. For me, that was not acceptable, so I willingly did my part by paying the credit cards off with my savings. Now, since we were off to a fresh start financially, I took a deep breath and, with a wink and a smile, I was persuaded we could anticipate a bright future ahead of us!

Soon after our wedding, my parents started going to another church. Larry and I remained where we'd been attending together since I returned home from school. The pastor of that church had married us, and we felt at home there. I was playing the piano for worship, and Larry was playing trumpet. The two of us began teaching the junior class together for Sunday School. I noticed and admired Larry's spontaneity with the kids, and they loved him. I was convinced we'd make a great team.

I wanted to be the perfect wife, but I found it quite difficult to live up to my new husband's expectations. I tried my best to learn, but I wasn't much of a chef, and Larry was an excellent cook. .... Larry also liked his shirt collars ironed for work, something I wasn't accustomed to. So, even though I had been a night owl, I started getting up early to provide his fresh shirt.

This lasted until February, when I started getting sick on a regular basis. The home test confirmed it.

I was pregnant.

> **"I know that there is nothing better for them
> than to rejoice and to do good in one's lifetime;
> Moreover, that every man who eats and drinks
> sees good in all his labor—it is the gift of God."
> Ecclesiastes 3:12-13**

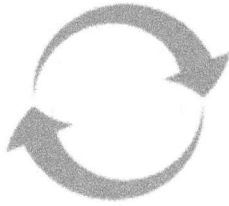

Chapter 6

The Honeymoon is Over

As you might imagine, morning sickness and the exhaustion of pregnancy don't make it easy to rise and shine and give God the glory, let alone to cook and iron for a husband. It wasn't long after the wedding vows when I asked Larry about reading the Bible together and praying at night; he responded by saying that I needed to take care of my own relationship with God. I was shocked. Devotion time was our binding factor, and I assumed he enjoyed spending those times together with me.

I agreed to continue working full-time until the baby arrived in November. Apart from being nauseated most of the time and feeling tired, I was very healthy and maintained a busy schedule. However, I found that Larry was becoming increasingly demanding and restrictive of my activities apart from him. I kept reminding myself that I was now married and needed to be sensitive and respectful of my husband's needs and desires.

During this time, I was invited to a Women's Aglow meeting with my mother. We went together to hear the speaker share her personal story of living with an alcoholic, abusive husband for 25 years. She described the way she'd prayed for and declared God's plans and purposes over him during those dark days. She continued speaking the promises from

God's Word daily, all the things she knew and believed to be God's will for him. She testified that after faithfully trusting Him, her husband was now saved and set free from alcohol. She was now experiencing a wonderful, loving marriage. All the things she'd believed for and declared years before, she was now realizing and witnessing before her own eyes. I remember leaving the meeting and thinking to myself, "25 years... I could never do that!" Besides, Larry and I had pledged our promise to one another for better or for worse. Since God had made it clear that Larry was to be my intended husband, surely that meant our future together would be bright, right?

Not too long afterward, Larry and I were finishing up our children's morning Sunday School class at church. I was preparing for the worship service when I was abruptly commanded by Larry, "Let's go!" I was stunned. I had no clue what had set him off. I questioned why and explained I had committed to playing piano for service that day and the music ministers were counting on me. I was told in a matter-of-fact voice, "I am your husband, and I say so!" So, we left. No argument, no explanation, no discussion with the pastor or ministry team, no saying goodbye to the kids. Nothing. Never to return.

Right away, we looked for and found another welcoming church outside of town, where we became involved and began to make new friends. Once again, we stepped up to work in the children's ministry, and I began playing piano. Instant commitment helped to ease the pain caused by our previously abrupt exit, but I nonetheless felt a sadness and an empty hole had been left in my heart.

I was aware before I married Larry that he suffered from mental health struggles all his life. He and my mom had an understanding with one another. My mom had grown up with an attention deficit, also known as ADD. I was familiar with the label but frustrated by it. I was reminded of numerous arguments in my childhood resulting from inordinate projects started and never finished. I had often heard my parents yelling after bedtime. This made me nervous, and I never wanted that in my family.

Larry said his challenge had been called "hyperactivity" when he was small, but now it was just beginning to be labeled as ADHD in the mental health field. He was also suspected of having a diagnosis called bipolar disorder. This is something I wasn't familiar with. All I knew was that he would blow up at the drop of a pin, say and do cruel things, and then be fine soon afterwards and think there was no problem. The best way I can describe it is that he was like a stick of dynamite with a short fuse. He'd explode, and everyone in the blast zone would be pelted with emotional shrapnel. People would be deeply wounded, but the post-bomb Larry would be okay.

Quite often, his blow-up would be so huge that he'd essentially black out and subsequently be unwilling or unable to recall the details.

If I attempted to discuss the matter, he'd deny saying or doing what was described and be angry at the thought of trying to work anything out. Conflict resolution was virtually foreign to him. As I was one who loved to keep and help restore the peace, this was hugely frustrating for me. I felt as if I could never anticipate what the environment would be like in our home. Larry was like an out-of-control ping-pong ball. I never knew which direction to plan for or where he'd land.

Another issue that exacerbated an already difficult situation was my default setting to placate and enable. As I mentioned, I was taught when growing up to serve others. I didn't learn, however, that it was ok to say, "no". This meant that quite often I did things for others that I didn't necessarily want to do. I also had few personal boundaries and often overextended myself, taking on too many projects.

I didn't feel comfortable speaking the truth if I thought the other party didn't want to hear it. I found it impossible to say "no" to people at church, planning committees, or to my husband.

Proverbs 29:25 says, **"The fear of man brings a snare, but he who trusts in the Lord will be exalted."** At this point in my life, I struggled with fearing man above God, and this was definitely tripping me up.

At the same time, I was beginning to discover that my husband's impulsiveness was creating new debt problems for him—now shared by me. He'd often make purchasing decisions without consulting with me. Since I was good at bookkeeping and finances, I was asked to take care of paying the bills, but Larry refused to stick to a monthly budget and didn't want to be held accountable for his spending sprees. He wouldn't discuss financial decisions and would open new accounts for numerous credit cards I was unaware of. He'd buy uncontrollably and then expect me to perform miracles to pay off his bills.

I became increasingly frustrated. I remember a conversation I had with God about my fears and concerns regarding money. I felt His reassurance that if I walked in obedience, my Heavenly Father would take care of me. My savings, investments, bank accounts, and even my husband were not my provider.

Despite these early struggles, there were still a few rays of light. My father-in-law seemed to take a shine to me and was quite supportive throughout our early struggles. He and my mother-in-law had purchased vacation property in Central Oregon.

They often invited us to spend weekends with them, which I enjoyed and looked forward to.

On one of these visits, Larry also decided to buy some acreage in the area as an investment and a place for future family camp-outs. I agreed to the adventure. We sought out a rural plot of land and purchased two scenic acres for a very reasonable price.

But it wasn't going to be just the two of us for long. "Baby" was right around the corner.

"When I am afraid,
I will put my trust in You.
In God, whose word I praise,
In God I have put my trust;
I shall not be afraid.
What can mere man do to me?"
Psalms 56:3-4

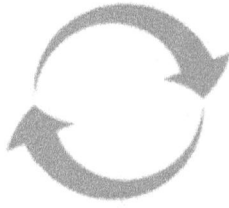

Chapter 7

WHERE THE RUBBER MEETS THE ROAD

Part of the marriage package is a mother and father-in-law, and I was blessed with two of the best. When I got married, I was told by my father-in-law, DeWayne, that if Larry ever mistreated me, he'd have him to answer to. Even though I thought he was sort of joking around, it made me feel like I had an advocate in the family.

Since I had a 1971 VW Bug, and Larry had a single-cab pickup truck, DeWayne was convinced we needed a more child-friendly car. He generously gifted us with a solid old-ie-but-goodie Dodge Dart 4-door sedan. Having received a suitable family vehicle, we promptly outfitted it with a set of new tires for safety and installed the required baby car seat for our anticipated trip to the hospital. Lucas Steven Hansen was born beautiful and healthy on Nov 16, 1981, weighing in at 8 pounds 5 ounces.

After his birth, as agreed upon, I quit outside work to care for our baby. I worked part-time jobs restringing pearls for the family jewelry store and also started providing childcare out of our home. The Dodge Dart was a handy vehicle for picking up and transporting children for short trips. However, since Larry would be home from work shortly after 5 pm, I asked all parents to pick up their children before then.

Sometimes, they'd be late, and this would frustrate my husband. Also, he'd be upset when the house was messy, and childcare wasn't the best job for keeping an orderly house. I would work hard to straighten up before he arrived, but no matter how hard I tried, it seemed arguments would quickly ensue. It became almost a daily occurrence.

Not too far into Lucas' infancy, we discovered he had a lot of food allergies and extreme problems with sensitive skin. No matter what we tried, his rashes got increasingly worse. Medical bills from the doctors, dermatologist, and allergist began mounting up.

Larry had little motivation for exploring new ideas or making new friends, and apart from a mild interest in electronics, photography, and fishing, he had very few hobbies. I would encourage him to try new things or "get out of his box", but he didn't appreciate my input. Often, when he was angry, he'd call his mom on the phone and have long conversations with her. She seemed to understand and had a calming effect on him, which helped restore peace in the house. That said, I always felt like there was something unnatural about him working his frustrations out with his mother rather than with his own wife.

The rejection and wounds kept mounting. Sometimes, I voiced my disappointments and frustration, but most often, to avoid conflict, I remained silent and stewed in my unhealthy thoughts and imaginations. Even though it wasn't my intent, a root of bitterness had taken hold and was beginning to grow.

Our financial situation was chaotic at best, though I'm thankful for my childhood example of financial stewardship, which guided me in matters of giving. My husband had made me responsible for paying the bills, and all the while, I was convinced that God was our provider. I'm grateful Larry allowed me the grace and ability to tithe and give to others in need when we had the chance.

Still, my babysitting wage was a lot less than my previous job. An extra mouth was crimping Larry's buying habits. One particular instance comes to mind in which he wanted a fishing boat. I explained we didn't have the money saved to buy a boat, but it didn't matter. Come the weekend, Larry went shopping for boats. He called me on the phone and instructed me to make my way in the VW with Lucas and meet him at a car dealer. When I arrived, he handed me numerous papers he'd already signed and told me to sign them all. I asked what I was signing. He informed me that he was selling the Dodge Dart for $400.00 so he could buy himself a boat. I responded that it was our family car and the only way to transport the kids. He gave me a killing look in front of the salesman and demanded me to "sign it!"

I don't know how the sale was explained to my father-in-law. I never talked to him or others about my personal conflicts. I didn't speak to family, friends, or people at church. I just cried out loud a lot to God. Somehow, I had the idea that if I were truthful to others about my private life, it would be the same as gossiping or being unsubmissive. The devil was having a heyday and just feeding me the big lie to keep me silent, isolated, and in the dark. This left me sad, frustrated, and lonely.

Another vivid example of rejection came in the form of a dinner. One day, I decided to try a special meal for Larry. I bought salmon and looked up an appetizing recipe in a cookbook. I set about to prepare a wonderful reception for my husband's arrival home from work. The children had all left daycare that day at their scheduled departure time, and I had set the table anticipating Larry's arrival, hoping he'd be pleased. Instead, he arrived home late, grumpy and irritable. When informed of my dinner surprise, he announced that he wanted to go out to eat. I detailed my time invested in the meal. No matter; he didn't want salmon. He wanted steak. My heart sank. So much for trying.

To add fuel to the flames, shortly afterward, I found I was expecting another child. As I no longer had a family vehicle, it was difficult to travel to our out-of-town church. We began attending a wonderful local church right behind our house. I was also attending a women's group during the week, which I believe was vital to my sanity, but sadly—and to my detriment—I still didn't open up or share my private life with anyone.

Days turned into weeks, weeks into months. Arguments continued. When I felt verbally attacked, my first response was to try to defend myself and argue back. Sometimes I would just be hurt and give Larry the silent treatment, but I was determined to make things work. I was excited about the new life coming. I had chosen the name for Lucas. So, Larry was going to name the next baby. She weighed in at 9 lbs. 6 oz. and was beautiful! I had always thought I wanted three children, but Larry wanted no more than two. He insisted I have a tubal ligation with the birth. I said we needed to wait in case something unexpected happened. He agreed.

That is until February. Life continued to be stressful. I didn't want it this way. I knew that God didn't want it this way, either. I also knew ours was a toxic environment for children to be raised in. I agreed to the operation.

It was about this time that Larry's paternal grandmother passed away. We inherited her Plymouth Valiant, so once again, we had a family vehicle.

I continued to babysit in our home. Larry now had two children to share my attention with, and I was often tired and lacked the energy or interest in evening romance.

Larry ruled the roost with an iron fist. When he had his mind set on a direction, there was little room for dialogue. Often, I wasn't in agreement with his reasoning, and this filled the atmosphere in our home with strife and frustration. I had always been a person who loved peace, and my goal was to find a road to forgiveness and reconciliation. When arguments arose with Larry, however, it seemed there was no way to compromise. It was "his way or the highway."

Proverbs 15:1 says, **"A gentle answer turns away wrath, but a harsh word stirs up anger."** I wish I had known how to practice this truth earlier. I know my tone of voice was not tender. Resentment had been creeping in. The atmosphere in our home was tense and critical. Larry's irritability seemed to be escalating. Each day, he'd come home from work and the arguments would resume. Larry complained that he was tired all the time because of crying kids. He seemed less interested in attending church and called me a hypocrite for my routine involvement. On top of this, I didn't measure up to Larry's expectations for housekeeping, cooking, or cleaning. Accusations were thrown around, and Larry started calling me "good for nothing" as a wife.

One Saturday morning, as Larry was preparing for work, the cruel words started up again. He spewed out the report that I used to be sexy, but that lately, the only thing I was any good for was bearing children, and now I wasn't even good for that. I definitely was worthless for sex.

I responded that sex was supposed to be an act of love, and what woman in her right mind would want to have sex with a man who treated her the way he did? Larry retorted that sex was my wifely duty. I argued that it wasn't a duty. Shoving me into the nearby spare bedroom, Larry told me that he'd show me what my duty was. Tearing off my bathrobe, he pushed me backward onto the bed. I was in shock as he dropped his suit pants and forced his weight upon me. He secured my hands above my head as I pleaded with him not to do this. I remember the warm tears rolling down my left arm as my head was turned away in disbelief. I was numb. I don't know how long it lasted, but when he got up and reorganized his business trousers, he left for work with the concluding comment, "Well, I guess you're still good for something after all!"

The trauma kicked me into some type of self-propelling survival mode. I must have called the neighbor across the street to stay with the kids. All I knew was that I had to talk to someone. I remember my tears mixing with some light rain falling on my face as I stumbled toward our little church. When I arrived, the back door was open, but no one was in sight. I went to the prayer room behind the sanctuary. It was dark. I left the light off as I fell to my knees, shouting out loud, "It isn't fair! This is not how it is supposed to be!"

Although my eyes were closed, immediately in my mind's eye, I saw the cross lit up with Jesus hanging in agony and pain, bearing my sin as well as everyone else's. He was alone and abandoned and also had tears running down His face, though mingled with sweat and blood. I heard Him sympathetically say, "I know."

In a moment, my perspective changed from anger and confusion to thankfulness. Time stood still as I praised God for His sacrifice and thanked Jesus for His willingness to pay the price for me, as I told God I wanted to and needed help to forgive Larry. In my mind, I rehearsed the plan to welcome him home after work. I was prepared for a discussion of offering my forgiveness instead of unkind words.

That evening, when he arrived home from work, nothing was said. All resumed as normal as if there were nothing to talk about. The incident was never brought back up.

"When they came to the place called The Skull,
there they crucified Him and the criminals,
one on the right
and the other on the left.
But Jesus was saying, 'Father, forgive them;
for they do not know what they are doing.'
And they cast lots,
dividing up His garments among themselves.
And the people stood by, looking on.
And even the rulers were sneering at Him, saying,
"He saved others; let Him save Himself
if this is the Christ of God, His Chosen One."
Luke 23:33-35

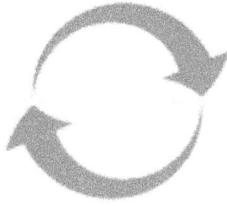

Chapter 8

A Bridge Over Troubled Waters

It was the summer of 1984. I was 23 years old, married, and had two children.

Now that I had a family of my own, I was becoming aware of some not-so-healthy patterns and habits that had been passed down from my parents. My mother was very concerned about anything and everything that might happen, and she was very careful to plan ahead for the worst. This tendency toward fear passed down to me, and I found myself also trying to control my environment and protect my children from all the evils of life.

I continued offering child day care in my home for two more years until my father-in-law decided to retire. He offered the family business to my husband, but instead, Larry decided to start his own business as an on-the-road salesman. Whenever Larry left town, I had a difficult time sleeping. After locking the windows and making sure the house, doors, and property were secured, I would still jump up to check each time I heard an unexpected noise. Since I never expected to be sexually assaulted by my own husband, the devil took full advantage of the trauma, adding to my already difficult struggle with fear. My personal anxiety kept me in a place of isolation and shame. The devil continually whispered his ugly lies into my mind. I thought no one in the church would understand, and even if they did, it'd be wrong to hang my dirty laundry out for others to see. Besides, I believed it'd be selfish to talk about myself. I should just stay silent and think of others. I didn't realize my own woundedness was actually preventing me from being effective in ministering to others.

After retirement, Larry's parents decided to sell their vacation property and purchase a motor home to travel. They began going south for the winters and, shortly after, decided to buy a home in Mesa, Arizona. We now had less family input into our marriage relationship and less bonding time for the grandkids.

Due to his distractibility and impulsiveness, Larry's job on the road didn't turn out to be very profitable for either himself or our family. Larry would always find "good deals" while he was out and about. He'd hide his spending habits, and our credit card bills again mounted up. Because of his lack of time management and accountability, there were downtimes that allowed Larry to give in to the temptations on the streets of Portland. This brought added doubt and conflict into our marriage. Hidden receipts and credit card bills proved suspicious activity. My dreams were shattered; I wanted to, but I could no longer trust. When he was home, the abuse continued, mostly verbal. I found myself questioning if there was any love in our relationship at all. The only thing that kept me committed and determined to make things work was remembering the YES answer God had given when I asked Him about marrying Larry.

One thing was certain: Larry didn't mind being waited on. In fact, after a long day at work, he felt it was an entitlement. He'd usually arrive home, kick back in his recliner, watch TV, and often talk on the cordless phone; then he'd shout at me across the house to come hang the phone up on the receiver. All too often, I was the faithful wife who jumped at his every beckoning call. Sadly, our children also learned to summon me from across the house. Somehow, it never occurred to me to say, "No."

One day I remember taking care of something upstairs when I heard Larry making a huge commotion downstairs. He was screaming and yelling about something, so I hurried down the stairs to hear cursing and expletives. I asked him to calm down and to watch his language. This seemed to escalate the situation, and he continued throwing blame and accusations. Back then, I didn't fully understand that we have an enemy who is always trying to divide relationships.

It says in Ephesians 6:12 **"Our struggle is not against flesh and blood, but against the rulers, against the powers, against the world forces of this darkness, against the spiritual forces of wickedness in the heavenly places."** I knew the devil wanted marriages to fail, but at times, it seemed like we were one another's enemies.

I wasn't in a place of trusting others for good advice or counsel in my life, yet I felt it was my duty to calm my husband down. Proverbs 15:18 says, **"A hot-tempered man stirs up strife, but the slow to anger calms a dispute."** In a not-so-soft tone of voice, I informed Larry that he was being unkind and unloving. My words seemed to exacerbate the situation. I told him his actions weren't godly and that he was sinning by his behavior. Larry's response was that he didn't care. His words stopped me in my tracks and cut to the deepest level of my heart. If Larry didn't care about hurting me, that was one thing, but if he didn't care about hurting God, that was a matter of life or death. Proverbs 15:10 says, **"Grievous punishment is for him who forsakes the way, he who hates reproof will die."** Larry may have infuriated me at times, but I surely didn't want him to die!

Time kept ticking ahead. Although I did everything in my power to forgive, every time we argued, I heard the recorded message replay in my head: "Well, I guess you're still good for something after all!" Almost daily, this message haunted me. Each time I tried to tell God—and myself—that I forgave, the pain was still as real and raw as the day it was spoken. At that point in time, I wasn't aware of all the ways the trauma was impacting me. I felt as if I were sinking into a dark pit of despair. I longed for human input and fellowship but continued listening to the lies of the enemy, who succeeded in keeping my secret and hurt in the dark.

Often, I found myself in a place of hopelessness and self-pity but would find comfort in the Psalms of David. I felt as if I could relate to his struggles and pain. Psalms 9:10 says, **"Those who know Your name will put their trust in You, for You Oh Lord, have not forsaken those who seek You."** Another of my favorite go-to Psalms was chapter 27, which is full of so many promises. It assured me that in the middle of conflict, God was my safe place and my defense. I received so much comfort in this, and I knew somehow that God saw, cared, and understood.

I often prayed for Larry after he'd left for work—mostly for God to change his heart and actions. A good part of the time I was really feeling sorry for myself, but also for our children. I couldn't see or recognize the part I was playing in enabling the turmoil or my lack of standing up for what was right. I was blind to my own ugliness.

One day, I found myself reading from Proverbs Chapter 1. I was captivated by the importance of wisdom and the benefits it brings to the lives of those who seek its fruit. The words from verse 3 jumped out from the pages: **"Righteousness, justice and equity."** I especially meditated on the significance of equity: something of extreme value that challenges a person to take their time and energy to invest in it. Patience is needed to see it grow, blossom, and hopefully mature into a massive yield or harvest. At that moment, I realized that if I continued to hope, believe, and pray, one day I would see the reward in my marriage.

New determination opened me up to repeated pain, as over

time, nothing seemed to change, and the 'good for nothing' ticker-tape continued playing in my head. It seemed as if all my efforts were getting me nowhere. I was exhausted and frustrated, just going in circles and finding myself back where I began. I often felt sorry for myself.

One day, during a session of self-pity, I had a vision. I saw a window into what Larry's life could have been had he married a former girlfriend. I saw that she had lost patience and divorced him. I saw Larry unshaven and drunk with alcohol. He was slumped back in a seat of depression, with no self-motivation. My initial reaction was to understand why she had given up on him, but then my feelings shifted to sympathy for Larry. I became grateful that he had not married her. My prayer shifted focus to asking God for the grace to continue loving Larry.

At the same time, I began asking for my husband's healing. I truly believed that God could and wanted to heal. I knew that healing from mental illness was no more difficult for God than any physical ailment. I believed It was God's will for Larry to be completely whole, and I prayed regularly for a miracle.

Then in 1985, we were offered the opportunity to go to a Marriage Encounter. I quickly signed us up. Larry's brother offered to watch the kids. I explained it to Larry as a weekend away alone, which he was thrilled about. When we arrived, however, he felt tricked and angry.

Thankfully, God helped smooth things over, and we both took the weekend seriously, following the given instructions and investing in the opportunity to communicate openly with one another. I had hoped to have the courage to discuss the abuse with Larry and seek healing, but it never transpired. However, during our time together, Larry was able to be honest about his mental health struggles. He described his traumatic birth, when his mother was over-sedated, and how this impacted his brain function. He was taken to a specialist at a young age, where he received a series of brain scans. His parents were told by the doctors that he needed medication to calm his mind and body to function normally. They informed his mother that raising Larry would require the same energy and effort as raising ten boys. Larry was put on medications at age five, but when he began school, he was teased by other kids. This led him to hide his medications. Larry recounted the times he was blamed for misbehaviors in the classroom. He recalled one time when his teacher was writing on the blackboard, and laughter broke out. The teacher turned around, rushed immediately to Larry's desk, picked him up by the shirt, and dragged him to the hallway. He was left there alone with a crushed heart and torn shirt. What's more, he said he wasn't even the one to blame.

This type of story was repeated throughout his childhood and youth. He was born with a smirk on his face, and this made him a target for punishment. As a result, Larry would turn to his mother for comfort. She had a soft spot in her heart for him, and because she felt responsible for his lack of oxygen at birth, she sometimes made excuses for his behavior to compensate for her guilt. Larry also believed the medication had stunted his growth, as he grew only to a height of 5'3". He felt he was inferior to others because he could never see out or over the crowd. Believing years ago that children grew out of the "hyperactivity," Larry discontinued taking meds after his sophomore year of high school.

During this marriage seminar, Larry was successful in describing his shortcomings, and I gained a better understanding and developed added compassion. We prayed together and took the time to remember the qualities we first appreciated in one another. Larry was one of the most generous individuals I knew. He was a hard worker and did his best to provide for his family. He had a good work ethic and was honest. He was kind to the elderly and had great respect for his parents and mine.

I did learn a truth that weekend that changed me for the good. I discovered that love isn't a feeling or an emotion. It's a decision. A choice. An action. I had chosen to and would continue to love my husband. We returned home with a renewed commitment to one another and to our marriage. My hope was restored, and once again I believed that God would use us as a couple toward the mission vision He had placed in my heart.

"He is the Lord our God;
His judgments are in all the earth.
Remember His covenant forever,
the word which He commanded
to a thousand generations.."
1 Chronicles 16:14-15

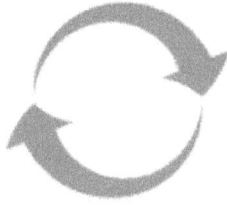

Chapter 9

So Quickly Forgotten

When I was a girl, it was fun to put on a princess dress and dream and fantasize about knights riding on white horses. I think it's natural to carry just a little bit of those hopes for real-life fairy tales into adulthood. But in real life, frogs don't turn into princes, and God isn't a genie who grants our every wish. In reality, fairy tales don't come true. Similarly, I also found that Marriage Encounters aren't a quick fix. Words, even with good intentions, can seem cheap, and promises can easily be forgotten. Relationships can be exhausting, and they take a lot of seriously hard work.

We'd returned home to our two young children, work, bills, and the familiar fuss. But Larry was not on medication. I still had no one to be accountable to, and commitments were easier said than done.

During the day, I tried to be the loving mom that our kids needed. I continued attending my women's group. Our children were making friends there and at church. I still hadn't been able to trust anyone to share my personal struggles at home. I found myself conflicted regarding my spiritual goals, and my secrets remained hidden in the dark.

We found it difficult to stay on top of our financial obligations. By this time, we had taken out personal loans from our family, applied for our own personal loans, and participated in debt consolidation programs. I didn't know what to do. I cried out to God. He was faithful. After receiving an anonymous gift of food left on our porch, it was decided in the summer of 1986 that I would return to work with a regular paycheck and medical insurance for our family. Since I had worked as a pharmacy technician for a department store prior to our marriage, I returned to work for the retail chain once again. I maintained evening schedules so Larry could stay home with our kids at night. Shortly after my return to work, Larry also decided to abandon his self-employment job and return to retail work. He had several years of management experience, as well as a lot of jewelry know-how from working for his parents. So, he decided to apply as a manager at the department store in the jewelry department, a position for which he was promptly hired. He was dedicated, worked hard, and was promoted quickly.

However, in his personal life, things weren't going so well. He didn't have close friends. I tried to encourage relationships outside the home, but often, after agreeing to events or get-togethers, he wouldn't feel well, and our plans would fall through. His mother had long suffered with a sensitive colon, and now Larry would cite this inherited illness to excuse himself from activities. We would plan and promise outings with the kids, but at the last minute, he'd change his mind, reporting he wasn't feeling well. In our earlier years together, I would also cancel my plans to stay behind with Larry, but this had become such a common occurrence that I now began to keep my commitments and go without my husband, often making excuses to the hosts.

Though this malaise was a usual preclusion to gatherings, there were also a few exceptions. For instance, one day, I was delighted to be contacted by Kari, one of my closest friends prior to marriage and a bridesmaid in our wedding. She was now married herself and had a new baby. It'd been years since we'd seen one another, and I was thrilled to reconnect. Our family was invited over for dinner and games to meet her husband, James, and their new baby. I was excited to catch up, share memories, and build new ones. I had optimistically thought that perhaps our friendship would be rekindled, our husbands would hit it off, and our kids would build meaningful, lasting relationships.

The meal was enjoyable, and it was great fun introducing our children to one another. Kari and I loved playing Pinochle together as teenagers, so it was natural to want to continue the tradition with our husbands. So, the games began. Larry wasn't familiar with Pinochle, but as with all games, he was very competitive. Maybe because of unfamiliarity, his voice became louder, his temperament frustrated. His words became increasingly attacking, critical, and rude. Finally, Kari's husband stood up and announced the visit was over. Larry wasn't welcome in his home if he couldn't speak to his own wife respectfully. No one had ever taken a stand like that before. It was definitely an intervention, but no plan of action was offered. No advice for change was given. I wasn't sure what to do. Had I asked for help at that moment, counsel may have been offered. But I was stunned and remained utterly silent. Sadly, we were shown to the door, never to be invited over again.

Battlefields and wounds marked much of the home environment, and discipline certainly was part of that. Even though our children were young, Larry had high expectations for them and punished them severely. Lucas was expected to set the example for his younger sibling, and when he contested the unfairness of his punishments, he was often told by his father to pack his bags and leave. This unfortunate drama played out numerous times in Lucas' childhood from age five onwards.

I remember many times praying with our kids at night while they were hurt or crying and reminding them of the importance of forgiving their father. At the same time, I could hear the recording repeat in my own mind, "I guess you're still good for something after all," and I would once again ask God to help me forgive.

As I mentioned earlier, I naturally followed in my mother's footsteps, and it was normal for me to live with a heightened sense of worry. Going to work and leaving our children in the evenings was causing my fear and anxiety to go through the roof. I knew how distractible Larry was, and I wasn't confident in his ability to care for our two little ones alone. Then, one week, a speaker was invited to our church for a conference targeting fear. I was quick to enroll.

In this conference, I learned that magnifying fear is really believing our imaginations to be greater than God and His abilities. This is what the enemy wants us to believe, but it's a total lie. At the moment this truth was revealed, I understood and repented and was set free. I fell to the floor under the mighty power of God's Holy Spirit and lay there while God ministered to me His truth and deliverance. During this time, God confirmed that He hadn't forgotten the vision He'd placed in my heart for missions. I didn't know how or when, but I believed God. What an amazing and liberating experience. As a result, my way of thinking was drastically changed. I realized that God sees all, cares immensely more than I do, and never lets a detail go unchecked. What a burden off me!

In the fall of 1988, Larry was promoted to the jewelry manager of his own store. This meant relocating to Coos Bay, Oregon. We took a weekend trip to the coast and found a cute little Cape Cod home. The owners were willing to carry the contract, so we packed our bags for our first move as a family.

"The mind of a man plans his way,
But the Lord directs his steps."
Proverbs 16:9

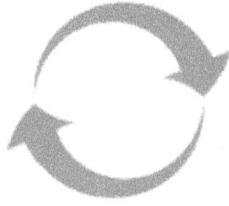

Chapter 10

HEADING WEST

We decided to lease out our house in Canby and, at the same time, buy a single-family home in our new community. I was able to transfer to the pharmacy in Coos Bay and continue working my evening shift for the same company. Our kids both had birthdays the following month and would turn seven and five. We started a home-schooling education in Canby and would continue with the same curriculum on the coast. Shortly after completing the move, we found a church close by.

Since Larry was a manager, he often felt that he needed to work weekends. I never worked on Sunday, so the kids and I could regularly attend church. However, when Larry did have the chance to attend, we once again started getting involved in children's ministry, and this is when we first became interested in puppetry. Our own children began learning the skill and enjoyed helping.

My husband's responsibility as store manager required long hours, which meant we saw less and less of one another. Quite often, I took the kids to the pharmacy with me to begin my shift and trade them with Larry, who would bring them back home. As Lucas grew older, Larry expected more of him and was increasingly harsh with discipline. Often, I felt the punishments were extreme and abusive, but once again, Larry stood his ground as head of the house, and his decisions were firm. This caused ongoing disagreements. I'm sure this also caused dilemmas for our children, as they were taught the love of God but often saw a different reality modeled by us both as parents.

When Larry was in a manic or irrational frame of mind, he'd have huge mood swings. Sometimes, he was motivated to conquer the world. He would start projects and insist we all jump on board to help, whether we were interested or not. He'd push us all until the job was finished to his liking. At other times, he'd come home from work and not want to be bothered by anyone. He'd tell everyone to be quiet and instructed the kids to give him an hour of peace. My confused ideas about submission continued to cloud my judgment about taking a proper stand or seeking help. I knew deep down that Larry had a kind heart and wanted to be a good husband and father. I just didn't know why he reacted the way he did or which way to turn. Satan had been doing a great job of continuing to keep me isolated from others, convincing me to avoid asking for input.

We were blessed to live close to the Pacific Ocean. Spending time at the beach was one of our favorite pastimes. It was a great place to escape the stress of our busy life and home. My children could play for hours, chasing our family dog, climbing sand dunes, and doing cartwheels. During those peaceful outings, I was grateful to be refreshed and could sense God's care and presence renewing my tired soul.

One Sunday, while Larry and I were attending a worship service together, the pastor issued a plea for adult volunteers to accompany the youth group on a two-week trip to Mexico. The plan was to drive an old school bus south through California, stay in churches along the way, and then head across the border to assist Habitat for Humanity in building two different homes in a slum area. While building, the plan was to do a Vacation-Bible-School-type ministry with the local children in the afternoons. Afterwards, the hope was to visit an orphanage, bringing gifts and crafts for the children and helping to paint the facilities. To my surprise, it was Larry who brought up the opportunity after the service and asked if I would like to go. If this were to happen, it meant he'd also need to take a vacation to care for our own children. Of course, I was delighted with the offer and excitedly said, "Yes!"

I was 30 years old, and this would be the first time I would be apart from Larry in our ten years of marriage. Our mission team started meeting to prepare for the trip, and before you knew it, we were off on a retired school bus full of young people. It took us two days to reach the Mexican border. On the way, we stayed the night at a few host churches where we were prayed for and given offerings and donations. We continued past the border, where we set up our campsite in a remote area outside the city of Tecate. The next day, we arose early to do our heavy labor before the heat of the day. We divided our team into two groups to work on two separate homes in the same area. In the afternoon, we began knocking on doors to invite the neighborhood children to our program. This is how the schedule continued. Diligence paid off, and both homes were completed that week. We celebrated with the children by breaking a piñata in each of the newly built homes and then blessed and bid farewell to their occupants.

Meanwhile, one of our teenagers stayed behind in camp. She had not been feeling well and was left there to rest. We were in a remote area with no phone reception, but one of the leaders successfully received a message sent by a family member of the girl. Someone she knew had come down with measles. Now we realized why our young lady was sick. She'd been exposed prior to leaving. At this point, her temperature was rising. We all went to prayer regarding our plan of action. We'd intended to head to the orphanage, but now we knew we couldn't expose the children there. We also needed to keep our girl cool. We felt led to move toward the coast of Baja, and Ensenada is where we found ourselves. In searching the area, we came upon Jorgé, a caretaker of a local church who agreed to let us stay there. As our team got to know our host, the girl—who was given a cool area to rest—miraculously recovered more rapidly than anyone anticipated.

The team had the time of their lives as Jorgé taught our youth the craft of leatherwork and how to efficiently crack a bullwhip. Jorgé shared the story of his wife, who was living on the mainland. She was nearly deaf and in need of hearing aids. This gentleman didn't have the funds to purchase them but had been offered this caretaker job. Though far away, he was saving money in order to return home and buy her what she needed. He had thought it would take several more months to save for the purchase price.

We explained our predicament to him and described the inventory we'd brought for the orphanage staff and children. We now understood that God wanted us to bless his community there. Needy parents and children were invited to the church, where we were able to give out clothing, toys, and school supplies. With the help of our host, we were even able to purchase and prepare a wonderful meal to share. Many people in the community were able to receive God's gifts with the cooperation of the local church and friends from another country. We had all kinds of extra donations. When we opened the bags, we found numerous pairs of eyeglasses to give out, as well as a set of virtually new hearing aids. We immediately knew who they were for. To make a long story short, our Spirit-led visit was the highlight of our entire trip!

We started the return trip home, stopping to lodge in the same churches where we'd previously stayed on the way down. The teens were excited to testify of the miracles they'd experienced first-hand. We all rejoiced together. I returned home with renewed enthusiasm and energy for being a wife and a mother. The following month, we received news that Jorgé had moved back to the mainland to join his wife and that the donated hearing aids were working perfectly. What a beautiful picture of God's love and foresight in providing for this couple in a way none of us could ever have planned. Once again, I was reminded of God's care for me, my family, and our future.

Subsequently, when Larry had time off work, I was excited that we could share in the children's ministry. We began attending puppetry workshops together, built our own puppet stage, and even invested in numerous hand and full-body puppets. The following summer, we drove to Mexico as a family. We ministered by distributing clothing in impoverished areas and performing puppet shows with our own children. It stirred an excitement inside my heart as I wondered if I would finally see my dream of foreign missions come to pass.

Then, as the summer of '91 was drawing to an end, my husband was once again transferred to manage another jewelry department, this time in Northern California. As a child, I grew up hearing all the horror stories of California. We'd cracked all the jokes about Californians coming to visit but not forgetting to go back to where they came from. So, California was the last place on Earth I ever thought I would move to. Always up for a challenge, I was willing to give it a try. We were offered an acceptable amount to sell our home in Canby, Oregon, but decided to keep our house in Coos Bay and rent it out with a lease option to buy.

We packed the U-Haul and headed 419 miles south toward our new adventure.

"The eyes of the Lord are toward the righteous,
And His ears are open to their cry."
Psalms 34:15

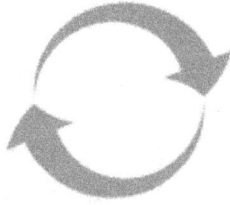

Chapter 11

THE LAST PLACE ON EARTH

Despite my negative biases, I had high hopes for our new location in October 1991. The move found us leasing a comfortable home toward the end of a densely wooded, pine-tree-lined, rocky escarpment of a highway. Although we'd come to settle near the town of Paradise, California, life wasn't quite heavenly. Our home was 2533 feet above our new place of employment in Chico. California didn't have pharmacy technicians like Oregon, so I transferred to the position of grocery checker, but I continued to work nights at the same store as Larry. A challenging new difference was the 35–40-minute commute for both of us. As we usually passed each other on the highway going different directions, we found even less time to see one another, and when we were together, the times were more stressful than ever.

The brief moments I shared with my husband continued to be filled with what we'd grown accustomed to: constant bickering, accusations, and attempts to defend ourselves. I felt I had done my best at being a supportive wife over the years. Even though I was always willing to share my point of view on how Larry could be a better husband and father, my advice seemed to fall on deaf ears and only added fuel to the fire. My dreams of being the perfect wife and mother were definitely not being realized.

We found a warm church family in Paradise. Although the pastors and parishioners were welcoming, I still never opened up about my personal life with anyone but God. I didn't take long in my new environment before I found myself stuck in a discouraging routine. Proverbs 14:30 says, **"A tranquil heart is life to the body, but passion is rottenness to the bones."**

Had I trusted and found the courage to encircle myself with a group of praying women to hold me accountable, I might have experienced the tranquility promised by God, but instead, I found myself stewing in the unhealthy atmosphere of my mind and suffering stress in my own body. Almost daily, that haunting, traumatizing message void of self-worth was replayed in my head from years before.

To save money on gas, Larry had purchased a brand-new, fuel-efficient Geo Metro, so we now had monthly car payments. It wasn't helpful that our lessees in Oregon weren't paying rent on time while at the same time damaging our property. Later, a former neighbor in Coos Bay offered to buy us out of the financial mess, so we agreed.

Although Larry was earning his highest wage since our marriage, the high cost of California rent, the gas, wear-and-tear of car expenses, and Larry's continued uncontrollable spending left our finances suffering. It felt as if I was on an uphill treadmill going nowhere. I had tried using all the tools I could find to get ahead, but I just seemed to be going around in circles. I would find myself back at the beginning with nothing accomplished. I was discouraged and felt like that 'ole Wile E. Coyote continually running into the face of a mountain.

I don't know if I was blaming it more on the move, living far away from my extended family, the exhaustion of raising kids, or my cranky husband, but I found my days increasingly filled with doom and gloom. If I had taken the time to reminisce, there really were many fun times and good memories shared by our family over the years, but honestly, in my mind, the bad definitely seemed to outweigh the good. Our children were growing up fast, and I felt guilty for the poor examples being set.

It had been twelve years since I committed my life to Jesus Christ as my Savior. Tragically, I believe the enemy of my soul had tempted and was succeeding in causing me to forget my vision. I had presumed on God over the years, and He had not come through as I had assumed. I wasn't cultivating an attitude of gratitude, and certainly, I wasn't aware of how much I was contributing to or allowing the negative atmosphere myself.

Proverbs 14:1 says, **"The wise woman builds her house, but the foolish tears it down with her own hands."** I had nearly given up on my hope for missions. I was living in the midst of daily frustration, self-pity, and disappointment, while my expectations for marriage weren't being realized. It seemed as if conflict resolution was an impossibility for Larry and me. I had tried faith, hope, and love, but hadn't seen the fruit I had dreamed of and expected throughout our eleven years of marriage. I had put my hope in a husband who hurt me, and the outcome was my offense and a hardened heart.

Since sarcasm had been my preferred humor, I was also quick to respond sarcastically with hurtful, curt digs of my own when unkind things were said to me. In an attempt to defend myself, my words could be sharp and cutting.

I'm sure my dissatisfaction in life was impacting our children, too. I really did believe the marriage commitment was "Until Death Do Us Part," and since I felt that death was the only hope to escape my misery, I began seriously considering and praying in that direction. At first, I began thinking and hoping for Larry to run his car off the road bordering the cliff on the way to or back from work. Later, I began to feel guilty for those dark thoughts and changed the focus of my prayer. I instead asked God to help me escape the misery, have mercy, and take me home to glory. Finally, I realized the self-centeredness of that train of thought as well, knowing our kids would be miserably stuck with a crabby dad for the rest of their growing-up days.

Then I remembered! The testimony flooded my mind of that woman years back who had declared God's will over her husband. God had honored her faith and set her husband free. Could it really happen? I was challenged by the words of Hebrews 11:6: **"Without faith it is impossible to please Him, for he who comes to God must believe that He is and that He is a rewarder of those who seek Him."** Would God work through the prayers of a frustrated but believing (or at least hoping) wife? I decided to give it a try.

My new determination and commitment to prayer changed my perspective and helped me realize the part I played in complicating the matter. 1 John 4:7-8 says, **"Beloved, let us love one another; for love is from God, and everyone who loves is born of God and knows God. The one who does not love does not know God, for God is love."** According to this passage, my thoughts and actions proved I really didn't know God. While focusing on myself, the devil was tripping me up. I was distracted from living the life God had for me. I wasn't able to minister to others properly. I couldn't truly bless my family. Years of offense and feelings of hurt and disappointment had crippled me. I clearly hadn't been walking in love.

I was 32 years old when our 12th wedding anniversary arrived. On New Year's Day in 1993, Larry bought me a NIV Women's Devotional Bible as a gift. On the inside cover, I penned in detail my prayers and declarations for my husband. I voiced promises, not just what I wanted, but what I knew to be God's will and plans for Larry—the good things that God wants and prepares for all of us. Even though I couldn't yet see a difference, I began to thank Him for the answers. Philippians 4:6 says, **"Be anxious for nothing, but in everything by prayer and supplication with thanksgiving let your requests be made known to God."** The interesting thing is that as I prayed and thanked God, I found myself changing. My frustration and anger subsided. My downcast eyes were lifted. I began to see beauty and hope. I discovered new things I enjoyed about the Northern California area and our church. I had a new appreciation for Larry, for his positive qualities, the effort he put into providing for his family, and his determination. As I invested in prayer and trusted in the One who never betrays, I felt as if faith, hope, and love had started doing their work...at least in my heart.

Meanwhile, things at work started to heat up for Larry. His district manager began putting pressure on him to increase sales and gave instructions to operate with dishonest policies. Larry continued to work with integrity. This led to an ultimatum that required moral compromise. Larry held to his conviction and high standards. This cost him his job, and he was ultimately fired in June 1994. I was on duty at the checkout and was able to watch as the store director approached Larry in the jewelry section and asked for his keys. I never admired my husband more than when I saw him leave that day with a great attitude, dignity, and a calm spirit.

The decision was made to move our family to the Puget Sound area in Washington, to live closer to Larry's brother and once again try his hand at on-the-road sales. I put in another request for transfer and was approved to move as a grocery cashier within the same company. We once again packed and loaded up the U-Haul.

Driving away from our beautiful Paradise, I realized that even though I never thought I could be happy living in California, I was actually sad to leave. The thought crossed my mind that if I could learn to be happy in California, I could be happy anywhere!

**"But thanks be to God,
who always leads us in triumph in Christ,
and manifests through us
the sweet aroma of the knowledge
of Him in every place."
2 Corinthians 2:14**

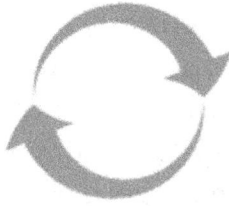

Chapter 12

ON THE ROAD AGAIN

Before school started for the kids, we settled into our new apartment in Kent, Washington. It was the first time I had worked a day shift, and I arranged to work while my children were in school. This was the 2nd time we tried public school. We had mostly homeschooled up until then. Our children had attended one year at a Christian School in Coos Bay and one year at a public school in California. Now in Kent, Larry made an effort to have coffee with Lucas in the morning and drop him off at the local jr. high school before starting the workday.

It was also a great opportunity for our kids to get to know their cousins better. Larry's brother had four boys. I had the privilege of babysitting one of my younger nephews often while my sister-in-law volunteered at their school.

While we each stayed busy in our new surroundings, Larry struggled with work. The world had entered a new era of technology, and my husband had no idea how to navigate it. By the end of the school year, Larry decided he might need to go back to school himself for some training. My parents had a large home in Vancouver, Washington, and after their generous offer and some prayer and ten months in Kent, we relocated once again to share my parents' upstairs living space.

Before finishing the move, our family planned a short camping vacation to relax at our property in Central Oregon. On most trips, Larry could be antsy to pack up and leave earlier than planned. This camp-out was no exception. The kids were enjoying every last moment, while he was pushing us to hurry up. The longer Larry waited, the angrier he became. I asked him to calm down, which escalated his irritated mood. Proverbs 15:28 says, **"The heart of the righteous ponders how to answer, but the mouth of the wicked pours out evil things."** Even though I thought my intentions were right, I often responded to Larry in a confrontational way. Finally, we were packed and ready to leave, but as he continued in threatening tones, I informed Larry that I wouldn't get into the car until he lowered his voice. His answer was, "I could kill you." He immediately picked up a boulder and threw it toward my head. I ducked just in time as the heavy rock bounced off the roof of our car, leaving a sizable dent. Both of the kids bolted from the vehicle and ran crying into the high desert. This left us alone for Larry to examine the new damage on the rooftop. We were still making monthly payments on our car, and now the paint job was obviously flawed due to his impatience. The lasting consequences of the hasty actions led Larry to recognize his dangerous behavior. He changed his tone as we went to search for our children, let them know all was well, and set off to our new home.

Larry enrolled in the Business Computer Training Institute in the fall of 1995. I once again transferred to the grocery section of a department store in Vancouver, Washington, and resumed working the night shift. Our kids both officially became teenagers and continued to take some classes through public school.

We were thankful to find a wonderful church home in Vancouver. As Larry wasn't working while attending school, we agreed to head up the children's church ministry for two services each weekend. We also began a puppet team and discipleship class for the youth. I was excited to work with Larry again, and overall, we were a good team. I appreciated his great ideas and faithfulness in serving, and Larry seemed to enjoy ministering with me as well.

During our time in Vancouver, Larry was a big asset for my parents around the yard. He helped with the upkeep and maintenance in his time off and stepped up to share household responsibilities with me. Larry always enjoyed cooking and BBQing and was instrumental in teaching this love and talent to Lucas. Things seemed to be a bit more settled in our family, and living above my parents helped to curb arguments in the home.

One weekend, Don Tipton, a guest speaker, came to our church and gave his testimony. He and his wife had begun a faith ministry in San Pedro, California, and ran it totally on donations and volunteer help. The speaker had written a book entitled, "Jesus and Company."[2] We were so interested in his story that we purchased the book that day. Both Larry and I fought over who'd read it first, and neither of us could put it down until finished. It made such an impression that we planned our next vacation to volunteer with the ministry.

"Friend Ships," as it was called, had several ships donated to the organization, and while staff and volunteers lived onsite, the cabins were designated as sleeping quarters. Stores donated and delivered food regularly to the port, where volunteers sorted and boxed meals to give out to the local community. Volunteers refurbished and restored usable donations of personal goods, vehicles, appliances, medical supplies, clothes, etc. These were loaded onto ships to be delivered to war-torn countries or areas hit by disaster, free of charge. It was all amazing to see and participate in.

Shortly after our arrival, we met a live-in volunteer who

---

[2]   Jesus & Company, By Don and Sondra Tipton, Via Verde Publishing, 1996

asked if Larry and I would like to meet with her during our stay. She offered to pray for us and speak into our lives. This was an interesting offer, so we agreed, and I looked forward to our time with her. Halfway through the week, a private place was found for her to share. First, she encouraged Larry as the head of our family. I don't remember the details, but it was very positive and uplifting for him. I was anticipating the same for myself. However, the messenger took a different tone with me. Instead, she admonished me on the inflection of voice I took when speaking to my husband. I could come across as critical and belittling. She challenged me to submit to Larry as unto the Lord and to take into account his counsel. What?! Obviously, she didn't know what kind of man I lived with! She didn't know the ways Larry had hurt me. How could she judge?

As she prayed for us both, I must admit I was defensive and harbored a bit of offense. Afterward, when I was speaking with Larry, he admitted believing the message was right-on from God. I wanted to be teachable and obedient, but this would all take some time to process. In the end, our time at Friend Ships made a huge impact on both our children and us.

Returning home, Larry graduated BCTI with honors and began looking for work opportunities. He had cousins close by who had a music shop and were looking to transfer their business ledgers to electronic records. They were excited to have Larry come on board as an employee. Larry enjoyed the job and was excited to bless his family with his talents. Lucas also became involved in helping out with the cousin's business. He had a keen interest in music himself. He began playing guitar and writing his own music.

In the fall of 1997, we once again traveled to Southern Cal to volunteer with Friend Ships. We enjoyed the intimate morning worship and devotion time together with volunteers. During a personal time of ministry, once again, I was reminded of God's faithfulness, care, and attention in my life and that He'd never forgotten about my mission calling, even though, at times, I may have forgotten about it. Our family had the opportunity to load a ship headed toward Honduras, recently torn by a Hurricane. Before sailing, the ship's captain needed to renew his license and make an emergency trip to Galveston, TX. Larry graciously volunteered to drive day and night to assist with his transport. The captain was able to make his deadline, and the ship sailed as planned. We were invited to come to Honduras the following spring to unload the ship, but Larry didn't have an interest. He once again gave me the "green light" to make the trip myself. How exciting! I quickly set out to apply for my international passport.

In the spring of 1998, I left my husband and children to fly south to Roatan, Honduras, an island of paradise, to help the Friend Ships team finish unloading the ship our family had helped to load the previous fall. I arrived on a weekend, rip-raring to go, but the crew was gone from the ship, nowhere to be found. I climbed up to the crow's nest for a view of the bay and spent time with my Creator. I found myself frustrated by the wait, as I wanted to accomplish as much as possible in my limited time there. As I felt my pulse racing, I realized a shadow was resting over me in the shape of a bird. Psalms 91:1 and 4 came to mind: **"He who dwells in the shelter of the Most High will abide in the shadow of the Almighty. And under His wings you may seek refuge."** I felt peace as I realized God was inviting me to rest under the shadow of a seagull! He made it clear that what pleases Him is not what I do but who I am. He wanted me to learn, even through a mission trip, that He didn't want me to miss out on entering His rest. It was a blessed week. As I prepared to leave, I couldn't help but wonder if Friend Ships might be the place for our family to serve in full-time missions.

In the meantime, Larry felt something stirring inside him. He shared with me that he thought he should be giving notice to his cousins to leave his job. I was full of questions. I just knew that God was moving Larry out of the rat race to fulfill my dream of missions. I set out to help him find God's will. I searched for opportunities in the newspaper, online, and in advertisements in church bulletins. I regularly asked him about his ideas on applying for all types of ministries. Larry reluctantly agreed to an interview with Teen Challenge but didn't feel the position was for him. I kept looking for and placing leads in front of his face daily.

Finally, out of frustration, he prayed. The way it was explained to me was something like this: "God, my wife is driving me crazy. What should I tell her?" He heard the answer, "Tell her whatever it is, you'll be doing it together." Larry gave me the message. So, of course, I asked for clarification. "Did that mean that I would resign from my job?" He responded that he didn't know. He just knew whatever it was, we'd do it together. OK, then. It was settled. I had peace.

In the spring of 1999, my parents made a mission trip to Hawaii, where they arranged to stay at the international Youth With A Mission base. Each day during their downtime, they were permitted to attend a session with a speaker, Fred, who was visiting from Colorado Springs. They were so impressed that they bought the entire teaching series to bring home to share with our family. The messages were life-changing for Lucas, who decided after graduation that year that he wanted to attend a Discipleship Training School in Colorado. It was the home base location where the speaker came from. Since my parents had such a huge heart for missions, they wanted to encourage their own children and grandchildren in ministry. They always offered to pay for our education costs for Christian school or mission training.

In further researching YWAM, I discovered that King's Kids was their children's ministry. I wondered if that could be the mission option for Larry and me. I remember asking God in the midst of my morning shower, "Is this what You have planned for us?" I heard plainly, "You can't imagine what I have planned for you." What could that mean? My heart pounded with excitement!

Lucas graduated from high school and submitted his application to the mission school for that fall.

Since moving south for the winter, my in-laws had been praising a children's home in Mesa, AZ, which had a choir that would routinely visit their retirement park. Larry's parents had recently gone to tour the home and were hugely impressed. They suggested we'd love it, so that summer, Larry and I planned a train trip to visit the home for ourselves and volunteer.

My husband and I left our two teenagers behind and boarded an Amtrak to Arizona. We disembarked at Flagstaff, where we rented a car and headed toward Sunshine Acres Children's Home. We were honored to be given a private tour by Aunt Vera, one of the original founders of the home and still full of vim and vigor. After showing us around numerous homes, we stopped by the dining hall, where Aunt Vera questioned us about our personal stories. When hearing about Larry's struggles with ADHD, she became very interested.

The week sped by quickly as we helped out in the kitchen and were able to spend time with several of the children. Soon, we were headed back to Flagstaff to drop off the car and re-board the train back toward the northwest.

The days that followed were hard to describe. Both Larry and I experienced the same phenomenon. Every direction we turned, we saw the children, thought of the ministry, and read Bible verses to confirm the vision. We prayed and made a commitment. If Sunshine Acres contacted us, we'd know. We arrived home and began unpacking. The following day, we received a phone call. It was from Gary Ingle, the director of Sunshine Acres. We put the call on speaker.

"This may sound strange, but Aunt Vera has been in my office every day since you left. She'd like to know if you'd be interested in becoming houseparents?" We laughed out loud as we described our trip home and our prayer, offering a fleece. So, Gary sent us the application. We applied and were accepted. We were scheduled to begin our new adventure on September 1, 1999.

It seemed as if Larry and I were making huge leaps and bounds toward good communication. I was beginning to trust him more as we had nearly paid off all debts, including his school loans. He promised to curb his impulse spending and discuss big purchases with me. I felt as if I was being lifted out of a pit of despair. Once again, my future seemed bright and hopeful. My prayers were being answered, and my husband and I were finally heading toward our mission call together.

I felt as if my heart would burst with excitement as Larry and I resigned from our "secular" jobs. Although it was not a third-world country, we were headed toward the mission field, and just as God had informed my husband, we were really doing it together! We began packing up to head toward Mesa, Arizona. Lucas was accepted to his school with YWAM to begin right after our move. It seemed as if, after nearly 19 years of marriage, my dreams and God's plans were being fulfilled before my eyes. It had been a long wait, but Larry and I finally seemed to be on the same page.

Then, in an instant, the bottom dropped out. I discovered my husband had been hiding some big decisions and spending choices from me. Once again, we'd need to make a plan for paying off a huge debt. Larry had been deceitful, and his lies didn't even faze him. He had no remorse. I felt betrayed. Not again! How could I ever trust him? I left the house with tears streaming down my face. Running down the sidewalk, I screamed out loud to my heavenly Father, "GOD, I thought I was finally starting to see light at the end of the tunnel! Now I feel like I am just going around the same circle again. I can't take this!" Then I heard His voice, as kind and clear as ever. "If I ask you to go around the circle one more time, will you trust Me?"

"Yes," was my resolution. "I will and I DO trust You."

"Hear my cry, O God; Give heed to my prayer.
From the end of the earth I call to You when my
heart is faint;
Lead me to the rock that is higher than I.
For You have been a refuge for me,
A tower of strength against the enemy."
Psalm 61:1-3

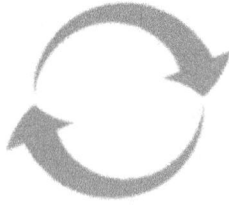

Chapter 13

HEADING SOUTH

Lucas was excited about the change; he stayed in Arizona just long enough to help unpack and welcome our first five boys into our home. He was aware of my heart for missions, and I recall a conversation he had with me before he left for his training. "Mom, I know you've always had a dream to be a missionary, but maybe God is going to let you see your dream fulfilled through your children." Hmm...Maybe that was how God was going to do things, but somehow, I still believed Larry and I would be more involved ourselves...and Arizona was a great place to start.

Sunshine Acres was situated on 125 acres of desert land in the heart of Mesa, Arizona. The property contained six homes, each with ten children, all of whom were parented by their own live-in parents. We were assigned as house-parents to "Saguaro Hill," where we were slated to parent ten boys, ages 5-12, in our home.

Every morning Monday through Friday, we'd get the boys up at 6 am for them to get dressed, make their beds, and go to our community dining hall for breakfast. During the meal, the founder, Aunt Vera, would read a missionary story to the children as a daily devotion and encouragement for their day. Then we'd return to the dorm, oversee morning chores, and send the boys off to school. Because many of our children were behind on grade levels and had behavioral and learning disabilities, we had our own on-site school where a number of our children attended.

Upon arrival in Mesa, I decided to start journaling my thoughts, prayers, and insights from God. I was amazed to see how Larry related to our new boys. They were all products of abuse and neglect. Many of them had been sexually abused, and most of them struggled with mental health issues and were medicated for treatment. Larry explained that he understood how they thought and could always stay one step ahead of them. His memories of his own childhood and being unfairly punished played into Larry's compassion and kindness toward our boys. Sunshine Acres was an amazing place, but we had never worked so hard before in our lives!

We didn't receive a large income as houseparents, but Larry and I did each receive the exact same wage, and I suggested we both take care of our respective expenses. As I continued to save, Larry continued to spend but, for the most part, was able to stay on top of his debts without my assistance.

Larry and I lived in our own apartment, connected to the boys' dorm, and we worked 24 hours straight for five days. We were given a break for two days off between 6 am and 10 pm, then back on duty for the nights. We'd still have our regular disagreements but did our best not to argue in front of the boys. We found ourselves exhausted each evening after the kids went to bed. There were often issues with the boys past bedtime, and Larry slept through only to find I had been up taking care of those who were sick or having problems during the night. It wasn't long before I found it impossible to sleep normally myself.

One morning after the boys left for school, I was sorting laundry when Connie, an on-site counselor, came in to talk about an afternoon appointment with one of our boys. During the conversation, Larry came into the room, loud and frustrated. He didn't seem to notice Connie as he proceeded to shout and throw accusations around at me, all the while speaking in a disrespectful tone. As he left as quickly as he came, Connie asked me if I was OK. I found myself making excuses for Larry, as was my common practice. I explained to Connie that Larry struggled with mental health issues and low self-esteem and was easily provoked, but I didn't take it personally. After Connie left, I pondered the incident. Why did I make excuses? I really did want change and, for years, had been praying for it. Had I possibly passed up an opportunity for help?

We drew upon our own parenting skills and past mistakes, as well as ongoing training provided through the children's home. Part of our requirements as houseparents was to participate with our boys in Sunday Chapel on the Acres. To build friendships outside of the home, we also found a community church where we met on Saturday evenings. Larry, the boys, and I became involved with activities there. I committed to a women's group, "The Well", that met weekly during the day. It focused on inner healing, and for the first time, I was encouraged to be honest with my personal marriage struggles.

As Larry's parents' vacation home was nearby, we would often go there for dinner on our days off. During these visits, they became more aware of our disagreements. One time, during dinner, my obvious frustration caused me to be bold in blurting out my feelings. I told my mother-in-law that it may have been easier in some ways to be married to an alcoholic husband rather than a Christian who acted like a heathen. Rather than offering advice or sympathy, I was shocked when her response was that God commands wives to respect their husbands. I needed to respect Larry. End of conversation.

Not long after this, Larry's dad passed away from an unexpected brain aneurysm. We helped his mom to consolidate her resources and move back to Oregon. We missed being close to our family and had a new appreciation for our parents. We said our goodbyes to Larry's dad and would now miss the presence of his mom nearby.

Larry began to feel comfortable with the daily routine and slowly let his guard down. One day, while the boys were doing morning chores, he became frustrated and started yelling at them. I had seen this many times with our own children but never anyone else's. Larry had lined them up against the wall military-style and was emotionally abusing them. I panicked and asked God what I should do. He asked me in response, "What would you do if you saw another houseparent doing this?" I knew I had to report them. So, although extremely difficult, I reported my husband that day.

Larry's response was to write a letter and resign from his position. Instead of the Children's home accepting Larry's resignation, they suggested he participate in mandatory counseling for three months. Larry agreed to the terms and was assigned to a staff counselor, but he didn't believe he had a problem or take it very seriously. It did hold him more accountable, though, and the incident never repeated itself. Something did arise in me, however. I had stepped out in courage and witnessed good results.

Maybe I could work up the same courage to finally talk to Larry about the abuse years ago and find closure. I made a plan to discuss the subject. It was our day off. I asked some other houseparents to pray for our important conversation.

I invited Larry to ride with me to a park where I set the tone by playing a meaningful song on forgiveness. I proceeded to explain my frustration with continual conflict and the inability to discuss disagreements and find resolutions. Larry didn't understand and asked for an example. I responded with the rape 18 ½ years prior. Larry exploded, "You're crazy! What erotic romance novels are you reading? It must be some type of sexual fantasy you've dreamed up or always wished for. This conversation is over; take me home!" I felt sucker-punched to the stomach, nauseated, and lightheaded. I tried to explain and recount the details but to no avail. Larry couldn't hear. We rushed back to our apartment, where Larry abruptly phoned my mother. Still in a fit of rage, he reported to her my insanity while detailing the accusation of the rape.

I had never brought the subject up to anyone. I endured my pain alone all these years, and now the shame was being announced from the rooftops. This trauma was worse than the first. I had gained every ounce of courage, only to be repeatedly kicked and trampled emotionally. I would prove it! I called for a polygraph test. When I explained the purpose, the operator asked if I had filed a police report. I answered, "No," as it was my husband, and the incident was 18 ½ years earlier. "There was no limitation for reporting" was his answer. I declined to file a report. I learned the cost of the test was $200.00, so I scheduled it.

Larry was beginning to calm down; he knew I was serious. I was frugal with money, and he knew I wouldn't spend that amount needlessly. Larry asked me to explain the details of the abuse once again, which I did. This time, he listened. He said he didn't remember the incident, but he did recall saying similar things. He didn't admit his wrongdoing but said, "If I did that, I am sorry. Cancel the polygraph test." Not the type of closure I was hoping for, but maybe better than nothing. This was a small crack to open the door for healing.

As Larry was convinced I could use some help on being a better wife, he went to the Christian bookstore and gifted me a couple of books. One of the gems was titled "Boundaries."[3] Other than the Bible, this book made the biggest revolutionary impact on my life. I realized that when I said "yes" to the things I wanted to say "no" to, I was actually

---

3   Boundaries, By Henry Cloud and Dr. John Townsend, Running Press Publishing, 1992

telling a lie. I learned to take baby steps in being completely honest. I also learned that doing things for others that they should or could do for themselves was handicapping them. True love helps, not enables. So, moving ahead, when my boys asked me to tie their shoes, I told them I would watch or help them and then cheer them on. No more allowing others to yell across the house for help. How freeing!

Meanwhile, I continued attending and building relationships at The Well. Through a teaching there, I learned that I could easily recognize an overt spirit such as control, but didn't realize that as I fought in the flesh with my own reasoning, I was operating in the same spirit and giving permission to allow for it to continually affect me. I knew that Larry was very controlling, but I didn't recognize I was covertly participating in the spirit's hold. This revelation prompted the following journal entry:

> *April 21, 2003: "Today I acknowledge that I have cooperated throughout the years with the unholy spirit of bondage. I've always known that I hate its fruit but have not recognized that I was a participant, by allowing myself and others to be intimidated. Today I repent, understand and consciously turn away, another direction, to make a new start with You as my helper, counselor and guide. Please help me to take a stand in love and recognize the enemy and his tricks. I believe things will be different in me from now on. The change in my heart and responses will also make a difference in my family."*

Thankfully, with God's help, I was able to come out of agreement that day with destructive spirits and partner instead with God's plan to walk in new freedom.

Due to my lack of sleep after three years of houseparenting, Larry and I chose to move to our own apartment separate from the boys' dorm and change our role to "Relief

Houseparents." This meant we began at 6 am and worked until 10 pm in various homes but could now sleep soundly at night without distraction. We relieved the live-in houseparents for their days off and knew first-hand the struggles that houseparents experience. They appreciated the way we shielded them from the various distractions on their days off so they could get their much-needed rest. Larry and I found a good system of cooperation between ourselves to make things work smoothly as a team. He'd sort the laundry each morning, and I would wake the kids to oversee their morning chores.

After completing his YWAM mission training, Lucas decided to move to India. Our daughter moved into her own place.

So, essentially, we found ourselves empty nesters.

"I sought the Lord and He answered me,
And delivered me from all my fears.
They looked to Him and were radiant,
And their faces will never be ashamed."
Psalms 34:4-5

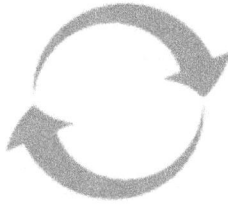

Chapter 14

Resurrection From the Rubble

Dr. Kelly was a counselor for many of our kids at Sunshine Acres. He came to the dining hall to share meals with them at times, and they loved him. One day, I built up the courage to corner him to ask if he ever counseled staff. He was very gentle and courteous with his reply: "Sure!" He had counseled several staff members. I asked if he'd consider taking me on as a client. He agreed and promptly asked when. I said I needed to ask permission from my husband and get back to him, which seemed to surprise the doctor.

Somewhere along the line, I adopted the belief that I couldn't make a decision without first asking Larry's approval. I had tied that into my confused idea of submission, and this had reinforced Larry's idea that spousal control was OK. Many times, it took all the mustering I could work up to ask permission for things I wanted to do or activities that interested me. Sometimes, it caused so much anxiety that I actually gave up and didn't attempt the request. This was way too important, though. I finally picked a safe time and worked up the courage to ask. Larry readily agreed and gave me the OK to seek counseling.

After confirming a day, Dr. Kelly and I arranged to meet weekly. As we became acquainted on the first day, I described the incident with the boys in our dorm and my decision to report Larry's abuse. After questioning me about raising our children and the environment in our own home, I was asked why I had the courage to stand up for these boys but didn't for my kids and me. I responded that these boys all came from backgrounds with extreme trauma and the abuse was not OK, to which Dr. Kelly emphatically responded that it wasn't OK for me or for our children, either. We're all equally valuable in God's eyes.

This was foreign to me. My counselor also interjected the fact that God is displeased with all aspects of abuse. After the first and greatest commandment, the second, as stated in Matthew 22:39, is that He commands us to love others as we love ourselves. If I allow or think it's OK for me to be abused, I'm not valuing myself as God does. He paid the ultimate price for my salvation and freedom. I need to recognize my immense worth before I can give that same love and esteem to others. I truly thought that I understood God's love for me and that I had a healthy love for myself, but I grew up being told that Jesus commanded us to die to ourselves, to take up our cross daily, and follow Him. This is truth, but I had a distorted view of what obedience looked like. I allowed the devil to devalue the child of God, whom I was, and I essentially became a doormat for others. How could I really value, give advice to, and love others the way that God intended? This was a huge revelation to me.

We discussed the importance of forgiveness, but that forgiving isn't the same as trusting. Forgiveness is given freely, while trust is earned and built upon. I also voiced my struggle with unexplained anxiety when Larry would come unexpectedly into a room, space, or building. I reported my deliverance from unreasonable fears in 1988, but I realized my continuing anxiety was tied to trauma from our marriage relationship. Dr. Kelly's insight and wisdom prompted him to give me the assignment of recording every time I experienced anxiety, how it manifested, how long it lasted, and to what degree it impacted me on a scale from 1 to 10.

It was shocking to discover how seriously my anxiety was influencing my life. That week, I recorded episodes several times daily with a degree of 9-10, lasting 15-20 minutes. Symptoms included a racing heart, sweating, fast breathing, stomach and chest tightening, and pain. I had no idea of all the ways this fear had affected me physically over the years, let alone crippling me from living out the potential of who I was created to be.

The following week, I returned with my data and felt ready to report the experience of my sexual abuse. Since I had never described the incident to anyone except to Larry earlier that year, I expected Dr. Kelly to gasp, make painful and sympathetic faces, and give responses like "Oh, no!" or "That's terrible." Instead, he listened with a non-responsive face and just wrote on his notepad. This discovery in itself showed me what was still inside, even after years of trying to forgive. The pain was as strong as that dreadful day back in 1984. My counselor then gave me the assignment to read the book, "The Bondage Breaker,"[4] the following week and continue to record my anxiety attacks.

Reading this book was another huge eye-opener for me, as it was made plain that true forgiveness has no strings attached. When Jesus was being punished for our sins, He stretched out His arms and said, "Father, forgive them, for they know not what they do." Period. Not if they're really sorry. Not if they know and remember all the details of their sin. Not if they promise never to do it again. No turning over a new leaf required. Forgive them, period. Wow! My forgiveness had several hopes attached to it.

In the latter part of Matthew 18, there's a parable about a

---

4   The Bondage Breaker, By Neil T. Anderson, Harvest House Publishers, 1990

servant who was forgiven a debt, but this same man wouldn't forgive someone who owed him. According to this story, the only time God won't forgive us is when we don't forgive others from our heart. It doesn't matter how many times we've been hurt. Forgiveness is the most important and powerful act of the will. It's not just for the one who caused the offense, but actually for the one who's wounded. Over the years, I had done all I could in my natural strength to forgive Larry but had always hoped that he'd understand the depths of my hurt and do his part to make things right. I couldn't do it on my own, but with God's help, that day, I released him from all expectations and set him free. I forgave Larry from my heart. In doing so, I walked into a true freedom for myself.

That week, we began our morning in the young boys' dorm. I got the boys up and sat down outside the laundry room, waiting for them to finish their chores. Larry had gone in to hang up the clothes, but to his shock, the houseparents had left a new puppy locked inside who had pooped all over the floor! I could hear Larry as he yelled, cursed, and shouted at the puppy. He also cursed the houseparents for leaving the dog and mess for him to step over or clean up. I was concerned that Larry might kick or hurt the puppy in his anger. I felt bad for the pup. Suddenly, I heard God say, "Larry is a barking dog." I had to stop myself from laughing out loud. I quietly told God that He was being mean, but I knew that He was being serious. Then, I began an argument with God, reasoning that His comment was not scriptural. The Bible talks about the devil being like a roaring lion, but nothing about barking dogs. This required a word search.

So, after the boys left for school that morning, I got out my trusty word-search Bible and looked up dogs. To my surprise and interest, no biblical dogs found listed were pets. Dogs were scavengers. They lived outside the city and were feared by the people. The amazing thing is that we need not fear. It's all filtered through our perspective. Larry saw the puppy as a nuisance and irritant. I saw the same puppy as an innocent little pet who wanted to please and be a companion but wasn't potty trained yet. When God informed me that Larry was a barking dog, He wanted me to know it was a matter of perspective. I could continue to be intimidated by the barking dog or have compassion for him. What would it be? The light bulb of revelation turned on. WHAM! Thank you, God! It only took an instant to receive the miracle of deliverance, and I was free. The rest of the week, I had no more records of anxiety levels to report, and Dr. Kelly was thrilled for me.

Over a couple of years of counseling, I was healed from many other unhealthy patterns and false beliefs I had grown up with. It took a while for me to feel comfortable by responding in new and healthy ways. Dr. Kelly kept reminding me to "not get caught up in the dance;" in other words, walk in the light of my new truth. When asked what I would like to do for myself, I realized I couldn't think of an answer. I seemed to always be invested in doing things for others. It felt selfish to think of myself. When asked what I would like if given the choice, I answered, "Ride a motorcycle!" So, at Dr. Kelly's advice, I started out looking for a motorcycle to purchase.

My trophy ended up being a 100-year-anniversary model wrapped up as a beautiful Harley Sportster 1200. I took a class to get my endorsement, and I was on my way to realizing a long-held dream of mine. The next thing I knew, Larry asked to go with me for a ride. How hilarious were the double-takes at intersections as viewers saw a man riding on the back! However, Larry complained that my seat was uncomfortable for him. We needed to go to the Harley dealer to buy a new seat. As I wasn't used to the added weight backing into the parking space, the bike tipped over right there in the dealer's lot. I was frantic as I checked for possible damage to my new baby. Larry inquired, "What about me?!" Then, the light bulb turned on, and I recognized the craziness of it all. This was my bike, and I was being coerced into buying a seat for Larry? Nope. No new seat. If Larry wanted to ride a motorcycle, he could get his own endorsement and save for a bike.

Once again, we were offered an opportunity to go on a mission trip with a team from church. This time, Larry was interested as well. We were to fly into the capital of Guatemala and drive up into the mountains to work with a local doctor providing assistance to a low-income community. Halfway up the mountain, we stopped for a meal. Larry was engaged in a conversation with our team leader and was hardly stopping to take a breath. In the middle of the sentence, he lost his train of thought and asked me to give input to complete details on his subject matter. This had previously been a common occurrence when we visited with others and was hugely frustrating for me. Now was the first time I had the courage to request, as kindly as possible, that Larry finish his own conversation. It took a while, but when reminded, my husband was able to change this habit, and I stepped into another new area of freedom.

Each time I traveled to another country, I could feel myself becoming invigorated and recharged in a supernatural way. During our outreach in Central America, I also sensed Larry's enthusiasm while ministering to the new people groups. I so hoped he would catch the mission bug permanently. Without a doubt, we both enjoyed our fantastic trip to Guatemala.

Forgiveness is a wonderful thing. It frees the forgiver. I could hear God's voice more clearly. Colors seemed more vibrant, and my outlook was brighter. Life was good. No more pain, only distant memories. My attitude changed, and my tone was gentler. Larry saw the difference in me and decided that maybe he could benefit from counseling himself. So Larry scheduled an appointment with Dr. Kelly's associate, Teresa. In their first session, Larry was assigned to read the book,

"Every Man's Marriage."[5] Larry asked her, "What if I don't want to read it?" Teresa answered, "Then I guess we don't have anything to discuss." She didn't pull any punches. It's good that Larry had a lady counselor, because each week, as they talked about the chapter, he asked in disbelief, "Is that REALLY how women think?" Teresa would confirm the truth. Larry continued his counseling with her for about a year. He tried to put her advice into practice and responded to me in new and kinder ways. Larry admitted that when he first met me, he was attracted to my independent and bold personality, but shortly after our marriage, I stopped speaking or standing up for myself. He lost respect for me. So much for my so-called "submission."

Our counselors suggested we trade for a session, so with our approval, I met with Teresa, and Larry met with Dr. Kelly. While speaking with Teresa, she asked what I desired in my marriage relationship. I revealed that trust was the most important. Someone I could relax with and be myself. Someone who was really interested in knowing me, who'd truly listen to and take into account my feelings, hopes, and dreams. Someone who was willing to give and take and felt it was worth investing in our relationship. Someone who loved God more than anything or anyone else. Even though it hurt, and I didn't want to hear it, Teresa informed me that she wasn't sure that Larry was capable of fulfilling all of my personal desires. I was putting unfair expectations on a human being. God can and does miracles, but she suggested I look for a true friend I could confide in.

When Larry met with Dr. Kelly, medication was discussed. Dr. Kelly revealed that he himself also struggled with mental health and medication helped him greatly. He gave an example of a person who had a pancreas that didn't work

---

5   Every Man's Marriage, By Stephen Arterburn and Fred Stoeker, Published by Waterbrook Press, 2001

properly; insulin could help that individual live a normal life. In the same way, meds can help those who struggle with mental illness. After some opposition and weighing the pros and cons, Larry agreed to try medication once again.

The following week, Larry and I met with both counselors. We participated in an exercise where we'd listen to the message of the other for three minutes, then the listener would reflect and repeat the understood message back. The speaker would confirm if the listener understood the intended message or clarify the message until it was correct. Then we traded places and repeated the exercise. After several tries, it was discovered that Larry was incapable of listening to and absorbing a message for more than 45 seconds. It was necessary to cut the message time down to ¼ of the normal time for him. This was eye-opening and helped me to understand why Larry denied past conversations. He was unable to retain long messages. Once again, I was reminded that God had His caring eye on Larry and desired to heal him. My determination was restored to fight for him and our relationship in prayer. Larry found a doctor and began medication again. What a difference it made, for the good.

Old habits and patterns were changing, and I was thankful. My journal posting from February 1, 2004, put it this way:

"Thank you for the opportunity of letting me be myself. I am trusting that through obedience I will continue to be liberated and be the person you created me to be... no compromise and refusing to bend to pressure to be what I'm not intended to be. To be real-no mask, willing to be vulnerable in a way to minister to others."

Even though we lived separately from the children on the property of Sunshine Acres, I still wasn't sleeping well at night. Larry and I needed a break and decided to attend our own YWAM school. In 2005, after praying and researching different locations, we agreed upon Argentina. My parents offered to pay our tuition fees, and I had saved enough money to pay our bills during the six-month training. We resigned from our jobs, sold some of our personal items, gave a lot away, and put the remainder in storage. After nearly 25 years of marriage, I was finally going to live in a foreign land and realize my dream of overseas missions!

"Who is like the Lord our God,
Who is enthroned on high,
Who humbles Himself to behold
The things that are in heaven and in the Earth?
He raises the poor from the dust
And lifts the needy from the ash heap,
To make them sit with princes,
With the princes of His people."
Psalms 113:5-8

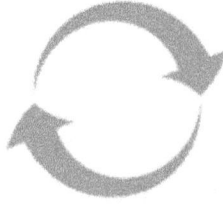

Chapter 15

HEADING FURTHER SOUTH

We arrived in Buenos Aires early in September 2005. A wonderful host family picked us up from the airport. For the next 2 ½ weeks, they were generous to share their home, delicious cooking, and culture. Larry was taught how to build a proper Argentine BBQ, and we learned to enjoy Inca-Kola and ceviche. After an official South American celebration for my 45th birthday, our new friends drove us to the YWAM base in Ituzaingo, wished us blessings, and said their goodbyes.

Our mission base was part of the University of the Nations. The Discipleship Training School (DTS) was a six-month course, the first required before continuing any additional training. I wondered if maybe Larry and I would continue after our DTS to work with children through the King's Kids program. I was open to and prepared for a new beginning for us, but I was honestly more hopeful for Larry to say "yes" to all God had to offer him. This was reflected in my Sept 28 Journal entry:

> *"I want to know Your voice clearly above the others. I desire this for all my family. Reveal Yourself to Larry in a real, personal way. That he would have an assurance and conviction of your leading."*

Although Larry experienced a lot of fear of the unknown and didn't speak a lick of Spanish, after arriving in Argentina, he really seemed to enjoy everything about it. He was like a father figure to the other students. They liked to mess with him, and he'd be a good sport and give it back. They were amazed that at our age, we would leave our homes, jobs, and family to travel so far away for this long a duration.

Most of the students were single and shared a room, but Larry and I were given our own quarters. The school day was filled with worship, classroom teaching, practical service, and homework late into the evenings. We shared meals in the common dining hall and built relationships with young people from every continent. We especially enjoyed sharing the biggest cultural bonding experience in all of Argentina, Mate!

Both Larry and I were assigned our own personal "Discipler," who was responsible for asking how things were going and being a sounding board and prayer partner throughout our intensive discipleship training. My discipler would meet with me regularly and ask deep and probing questions, which often nudged me out of my comfort zone. She'd challenge me to answer in new and personal ways, rather than the "Biblically correct" answers or to give the typical "religious" or Sunday School responses.

One of the first things we were taught in school was that we all have differences in opinions and ideas on the way things should be done. Sometimes, it's not a matter of right or wrong; it may just be a preferred way of doing things. Our culture teaches us specific manners of doing tasks, but it's not worth being stubborn, destroying relationships, or causing division. It's good to get out of our comfort zones and be flexible. We need to be careful and pick our battles. At times, it could be worth standing up for a matter of right or wrong, but otherwise, we might just defer to the way of others. This was a valuable lesson that I've carried with me going forward. "It's not right, it's not wrong; it's just different!"

Some of our teaching was intense, and even though I thought all was forgiven, I was challenged to go deeper. Journal entry Oct 8, 2005:

> *"Father, you know the thoughts that were going thru my mind this morning. I thought I had forgiven everything in my past, but there still were strong emotions when I thought about many memories i.e.; leaving LO Assembly, selling the Dodge, many issues of control. Do I still need to discuss these things with Larry? You know that often I am motivated by fear of reaction. This keeps me silent. But you have challenged me to live in the truth-in the light. Sometimes the light hurts-both Larry AND me. Am I willing to be hurt again?! I trust you - Yes, I know you've promised, but sometimes the answer takes SO long. Years? A lifetime? Thank you for Your presence. I want to hear Your voice."*

Even though God had told me years before that He cared more about who I was rather than what I did, I still had a good work ethic and loved to put all my efforts into a job well done. As a child, my father gave his nod of approval whenever I completed a task to the best of my ability, and somehow, I felt that God did the same. For DTS, I was assigned to the orphanage for my practical service time in the afternoon. I cleaned the areas that were often overlooked in daily chores. Others from my school were also placed there, but I could be critical of others if I observed they didn't make the most of their time as I did. I felt dignified in all I was able to accomplish during the allotted time. Often, I was left unsupervised, but I believed my work was unto the Lord as I scrubbed and polished. I was pretty sure He was smiling down on me with pride at my attempts to do my best.

We usually had 1 to 2 days off from school, and Larry and I would walk to the Internet café to contact family by Skype or take care of financial matters online. Due to my height advantage and longer legs, when in a hurry, I could make greater strides over Larry on a trip. On this particularly hot day, I was traveling at a rapid pace down the familiar dirt road. Impatient to get out of the sun and arrive at our destination, I turned towards Larry, shouting for him to hurry up. Unknowingly, there was a huge chuckhole ahead. In an instant, I backed into it, and my ankle twisted with a pop. I was brought to my knees in pain. When Larry reached my spot to help, I was unable to put weight on my foot to go anywhere. It was necessary to hail a taxi and ride to a travel clinic for X-rays. The doctor confirmed it wasn't broken, but I had torn a ligament in my ankle. I was instructed to stay off my feet for 3 weeks.

The staff and fellow students were kind and very accommodating. They helped me with the stairs, and I was able to continue with all my classes. Though excused from practical service, I begged for jobs I could complete while sitting down. It was humiliating, and I felt useless. My perceived reality was that I wasn't being productive or pulling my own weight. Our leaders advised me to rest and heal, but after lots of negotiating, they gave me some ironing jobs. As I sat and watched others pass me by, something stirred inside of me. It was an uncomfortable restlessness difficult to explain. Maybe an annoyance at myself for being so careless and falling into a hole, or possibly anger at God for allowing it to happen. Journal entry Oct 27, 2005:

> *"So here I am. Waiting ... trying to learn to rest. I want to understand. I want to believe, but it seems contrary to what I believe is right. It's not wrong to work. You say, 'Faith without works is dead!' There's a huge conflict inside me! Please surprise me. I want to believe and understand what is right."*

One morning, as I sat there watching fellow students pass me by, a young lady stopped and presented me with a pair of earrings. She bought them from a lady who did handcrafts. She specifically purchased them for me. I immediately burst into tears. Here I was in another country to bless others. I was unable to demonstrate my strengths the way I had planned. I could only sit and watch, yet I was receiving gifts. I didn't feel worthy. I had so much ugliness inside of me.

When my discipler came to encourage me, she could sense the struggle going on inside but didn't try to fix anything. She actually seemed to have a satisfied sense of calm about her. That night, I agreed to turn in earlier for bed. More than my swollen, sore ankle, whatever was brewing inside of me was exhausting.

The following day, we started the week with a new teacher. He began with the topic, "You must be Born Again."

**"Without faith it is impossible to please Him,
for he who comes to God must believe that He is,
and that He is a rewarder of those who seek Him."
Hebrews 11:6**

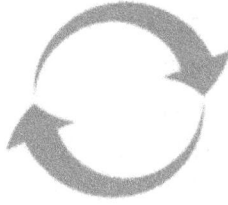

Chapter 16

A New Foundation

So, there I was, in the miserable state described in Chapter One. I was angry. My anger confused me. It exposed things inside I never knew existed and I didn't like. I became literally ill. I began crying uncontrollably. I couldn't sleep at night. I found myself arguing with scripture, with God, all the things I thought I believed. Larry was becoming worried about me. After a few days, he called two of my women mentors to our room to pray for me. Upon arrival, they saw me doubled up in the bed, asked me a few questions, smiled, and told Larry I was going to be alright, which confused him. They said a short prayer for me and left. I made a commitment that I wouldn't eat until I figured out what was going on. It was painful. It was messy. It was the best thing that has ever happened to me.

The only way I can explain it is that in the middle of my pain, God met me personally, and I was totally delivered from my stubborn intellect. The mind is a powerful thing. I had put a lot of trust in my upbringing, my memory, and what and why I believed it. I could argue my case before the best and usually thought I was right, but I was wrong. I thought I had every right to defend myself from Larry's attacks, and I knew it was my job to show him the error of his ways. God had allowed the foundation of my psyche to be stripped down to rock bottom. Now, He could rebuild, but on the proper foundation. Not what my parents said, or the best pastors or teachers. Not from doctrine, theory, books, seminars, or lectures. God did kindly assure me, however, that my former life hadn't been a waste.

Journal entry Nov 1, 2005:

"Well, I don't seem to have any answers, but I trust You and Your timing. Thank you for the time I was in the pit. I think if it did not happen to me, I would not be sympathetic with others going through it. I would have thought it was satan. Was part of it satan? I never thought such turmoil could come from You? But I praise You! You're AWESOME! I totally trust You and ask You to continue changing me."

I had memorized Romans 8:28 as a child; **"And we know that God causes all things to work together for good to those who love God, to those who are called according to His purpose."** I was assured that although I grew up seeing God through a distorted lens in many ways, He was happy to lead me into truth if I had a teachable heart. I saw God's Word in a new way. I was hungry and devoured it. It was life to my bones and inner man. I could hear God speaking personally in new and different ways, surprisingly, many times out of context, but still, His voice was clear, alive, and direct. I was receiving His Word gladly in my Spirit, not my mind. I saw 1 Corinthians 2:14 in a different light, **"A natural man does not accept the things of the Spirit of God, for they are foolishness to him; and he cannot understand them, because they are spiritually discerned."** I found myself letting go of critical thinking and judgmental attitudes. I was able to give grace to others like never before. I felt new, ready to trust like a baby. I've never been the same since.

There were several books assigned to us for reading material at school, all of them life-changing. One book that rocked my world was "Why not Women?"[6] My upbringing had implanted some wrong belief systems about women being involved in ministry, but the truths shared in this book shattered those false ways of thinking and the way I had responded to those whom God places in authority. God can and does use anyone who's teachable and willing to be used for His purposes. This includes young or old, mature or naïve, broken or healed, the downcast of society, those least likely to lead, man or woman.

I re-read a journal entry dated Sept 30, 2005:

"Do You have a calling on my life God?... for ministering to those who have been wounded? I want to know-I am willing-Please direct us & let us know in our inner being what Your will is for us. We want to be ministers of healing to others & I know that is Your will, but the way & methods we don't know yet."

Not long after my deliverance, we had a speaker named Wilson come to minister at our school for a week. He was from Africa, and it was his first time visiting South America. He was very sensitive, and when he wasn't teaching, he was watching and listening. I often went to class early and sat and prepared myself for worship and instruction. As I was sitting alone, Wilson entered the classroom. After a while, he came to speak with me. We didn't talk long, but he told me that God would be giving me a platform. I didn't know what that meant. I had never wanted or asked for a platform, but somehow, after Wilson gave me that message, I knew it was true. I didn't know how; I just knew.

Soon after, another thing that was impressed upon me was that God was a God of fairness and equity, and He was

---

6   Why not Women, By Loren Cunningham and David J. Hamilton, YWAM Publishing, 2000

offering that to me personally. I meditated on this for some time. My parents had taught me to save and build up financial equity through saving, investments, or property, but I felt as if God was giving me a promise that He was going to reward me for my investment into my marriage and family. I didn't know how this would play out, but it gave me great encouragement. One of the verses highlighted at this time was Habakkuk 2:3: **"The vision is yet for the appointed time; it hastens toward the goal and it will not fail. Though it tarries, wait for it; for it will certainly come, it will not delay."**

As God began to put me back together, He made it clear to me that I was responsible for myself. I could encourage others, but I wasn't responsible for them. Everyone is given free choice, and they're responsible for what they do with every choice given, just as I am. Journal entry Nov 17, 2005:

"Thank You, God! I am so blessed! I am SO thankful for Your faithfulness and continued work in my life. Thank You for setting me free and showing me the truth that I am not responsible for other people's feelings and reactions. I am only responsible to be obedient to You. What a load off my shoulders! I am free. Yes, I am saddened when others are upset and angry, but it is not my responsibility to take on everyone else's burdens. I need to listen to Your voice and if you say, "speak or encourage," yes, that's what I want to do, but YOU are the only one to take the burden. Yes, I will also pray and ask You to show me Your heart and intercede as You ask, but the burden is not heavy, because You take the burden."

Since our anniversary was approaching, one of the musicians at the school agreed to accompany me on the guitar while I surprised Larry by singing to him in class. It was a renovation of the original wedding song I sang to Larry 25 years earlier. That evening on December 6th, the teachers and students honored us with a silver wedding celebration in the dining hall. The following weekend, we were to set sail from Buenos Aires to Uruguay to spend time together, to thank God for His faithfulness to us as a couple, and to renew our 90-day Argentine travel visa.

As our theory portion of the class was drawing to an end, all of us students and leaders prayed about who would be on each ministry team and where we would go for outreach. Larry and I were invited to be a part of a team to do children's work in Patagonia. The plan was to cross over the Andes Mountains into Chile and return to the base three months later. We considered and accepted the invitation.

Larry and I were looking forward to celebrating Christmas in a new way, in a place where geese pulled Santa's sleigh instead of reindeer. We were excited to feel the warmth of the southern hemisphere and for our mission adventure ahead!

**"Now we have received not the spirit of the world,
but the Spirit who is from God,
so that we may know the things
freely given to us by God,
which things we also speak, not in words taught
by human wisdom,
but in those taught by the Spirit,
combining spiritual thoughts
with spiritual words."
1 Corinthians 2:12-13**

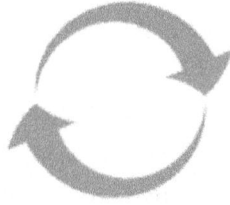

Chapter 17

JERUSALEM, JUDEA AND SAMARIA

Our outreach team was led by the young married couple who had discipled Larry and me during DTS. Neither had ever worked with children, so they were out of their comfort zone, but Larry and I were in our element. Those three months were filled with so many miracles, that it would take chapters to explain. It was summer there as we entered the beautiful town of Bariloche, where we worked with three separate churches to assist with needs in the community. We celebrated Christmas in a different light and found it quite refreshing, as the commercialism common in the Western world was nonexistent. We felt blessed in the spirit of the season to minister to a community that lived outside the city in the dumps. We helped with church leadership training and assisted with a children's Bible school in a very impoverished barrio.

Our input was requested, and our ideas were valued, as Larry and I had years of experience raising our own children, working in children's ministry, and being houseparents. During our stay, we slept in churches and in a community school where we were able to bless by painting and doing maintenance work. Through our efforts, some neighbors were touched by our service and ultimately became believers in Christ and part of the local church. I was paying close attention, listening, and searching with my spirit everywhere we traveled. I questioned God as to Larry and my future in ministry together but was cautious not to step ahead of God or try to force something in my flesh. Journal entry Jan 19, 2006:

> *"Proverbs 19:2 He who hurries his footsteps errs. God, I don't want to get ahead of you. I want to go the direction You lead."*

After two months of ministering in southern Argentina, we headed up the Andes Mountains to cross into Chile. When we arrived at the summit, it was necessary to exit our travel bus for immigration purposes. As he prepared to disembark, Larry became annoyed and began barking at me to carry his bags. I was sucked into the argument, attempting to defend myself. The heated conversation continued for some time, as I didn't back down from Larry's verbal attacks. Later that afternoon, our team stopped at a park for a picnic lunch. Larry's discipler, Jonnie, pulled me aside and asked to speak with me. I agreed, and we found a place to talk where Jonnie discussed the argument on the bus. He wanted to advise me against arguing back, even if I felt I was in the right. He suggested I let Larry run his course when he became unreasonable and allow him to bear his own consequences; otherwise, I would be in the same boat of foolish babbling and deserve the fruit of my frustration. At first, I took offense to Jonnie's advice but later was reminded and meditated on his words that were also clear in Proverbs 26:4-5: **"Do not answer a fool according to his folly, or you will also be like him. Answer a fool as his folly deserves, that he not be wise in his own eyes."** This challenged me to be thoughtful in my responses, and I was thankful for Jonnie's courage in approaching me over the matter.

Our arrival in Chile found us working for a month with another church, which again was requesting help with children's ministry. It seemed the entire outreach had been tailored to Larry's and my interests and abilities as we held daily clubs in the library. We built wonderful relationships with both the children in the local church and in the community. This opened the eyes of our leaders to appreciate the value of children in a new light and, amazingly, our disciplers, Stacy and Jonnie, discovered before the end of outreach that she was pregnant with their first child!

I had several opportunities to put our leader's advice into practice. When I guarded my mouth, I saw God's hand of favor and blessing. He affirmed His correction by highlighting His Word, Proverbs 10:19: **"When there are many words, transgression is unavoidable, But he who restrains his lips is wise."** Proverbs 29:20: **"Do you see a man who is hasty in his words? There is more hope for a fool than for him."** Proverbs 17:27: **"He who restrains his words has knowledge, and he who has a cool spirit is a man of understanding."** I was grateful for the Holy Spirit's counsel.

Daily, I was full of questions for God, pondering what He may have in store for our days ahead. I remembered the conversation with Wilson during our theory phase and knew my testimony could be a vehicle for setting others free.

Journal entry February 7, 2006:

> *"God, what does it mean that 'I will be given a platform?' I do know that if I am faithful in the small things, I will be given more. Forgive me for all the times I was afraid to be faithful in the small things. You are always faithful. I've never wanted or dreamed for a platform. If women or anyone else would be blessed or ministered to by my story, I am willing. I trust You."*

Returning to our base in Argentina, we reunited with other teams to celebrate all the wonders of God's faithfulness, graduate, and look ahead to future plans. It was clear that permanently staying in Argentina wasn't for us. Larry and I were both open to continuing our training with YWAM and decided to submit an application for the following fall to a Biblical counseling school in Chile. We said goodbye to our new friends and family from our DTS and headed back to the good 'ole USA.

Upon arrival, I believed it was a priority to speak separately with each of our children and try to explain my personal deliverance experience. Although I had tried to be a good mother throughout the years, I made wrong decisions that were motivated by intimidation. I had acted in the flesh through my lack of boundaries and misguided ideas of submission which had prevented me from taking a stand for their safety. In doing so, I had unknowingly contributed to the abuse in our home. I shared my desire to be led by the Spirit and asked their forgiveness in the unhealthy part I had played in our home.

Some time after arrival, we drove down to a children's home in Baja, Mexico, to volunteer and check out opportunities there. Sunshine Acres received word that we were back in town and asked if we'd consider filling in to cover vacations for houseparents during the summer. We agreed and moved back into the groove of relief houseparent duties.

One afternoon, I recall feeling disillusioned as I was riding down the dusty road in a golf cart toward the warehouse to pick up some supplies for the children. I had attended mission school with Larry, hoping God would bring my vision into focus and Larry and I would both have a life-altering revelation and realize our lifetime call to live out the remainder of our days in a far-off land, serving God and blessing others. None of that seemed to have transpired. Along the drive, I dared to ask this question: "God, I know you called me to missions. I believe you also called Larry. I've been patient through these 25 years of married life, but I don't see my vision coming to pass. God, I know I heard you clearly, but I don't understand. When I asked you about marrying Larry, why did you say, "Yes?"

I am not sure it was audible, but the answer was immediate and very clear. "I love Larry..." I knew God loves everyone. I was certain of God's love for me. He'd always been very close to me and faithful through good and bad, but I may not have felt like Larry was quite as lovable. He was definitely more difficult to love at times. But NO. God loved Larry deeply and unconditionally. Then He continued, "... and I trust you."

"WHAT??? You trust ME???" I was floored! "I am so NOT trustworthy! You are the only ONE who is trustworthy!" How can this be? My mind was flooded with all the ways I had failed throughout the years.

Could it be possible that the all-knowing, all-compassionate God of the universe may have said "yes" to the prayer of a twenty-year-old lady to assign her to an all-important, life-changing mission? Could it be that His eyes were intently focused on a young man who didn't know how to receive or give love, that He didn't want that man to lose hope or live out his life as a hopeless alcoholic? That God had orchestrated a beautiful plan to minister to that man and show His love through this young lady? That God knew she had the capacity, not on her own, but with His help, to be an instrument to show real love to Larry and give him purpose to live? Wow! Yes, it was true, and I had gotten it all wrong! I was flabbergasted!

Come to think of it, the very first relational conflict listed in the Bible was between brothers. When God asked Cain in Genesis 4 where his brother was, he answered back with a question, "Am I my brother's keeper?" God never promised that relationships, even in families, would be easy, but He did command us to love and forgive. If we don't, just like with Cain, sin is crouching at the door. Love and forgiveness are two of the attributes of God Himself. I'm not the only one who was given this commission. God entrusts us all to demonstrate His love, even when it's difficult. When we choose to offer love with God's strength, even sacrificially, we identify with Christ and are supernaturally blessed. That day, I had a paradigm shift. My heart changed. I repented and committed, with God's help, to be faithful to His important calling.

So, Larry was right those many years back. If I couldn't do a proper job in my Jerusalem, my own home, I wouldn't be ready for Judea and Samaria. There was still something stirring in my heart, though. I didn't believe missions was out of the picture for Larry and me. While reading Proverbs, this verse dropped into my Spirit. I didn't know what it meant but knew it was prophetic. Proverbs 24:27: **"Prepare your work outside, and make it ready for yourself in the field; Afterwards, then, build your house."** Journal entry June 24, 2006:

"I believe this is a confirmation that right now is the time to work outside & lay the groundwork in the field. It's not yet the time to 'build our house.'"

Not long after, we received our acceptance letter to the Biblical Counseling School in Chile. Sunshine Acres appreciated our work with the children and offered us a return position after completing our next six-month school, but Larry and I both knew that SACH wasn't our permanent place to settle. We finished out our relief position that summer and prepared to head back to South America in September.

**"Therefore, my beloved brethren,
be steadfast, immovable, always abounding in the
work of the Lord,
knowing that your toil is not in vain in the Lord."
1 Corinthians 15:58**

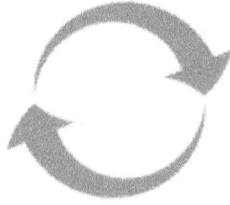

Chapter 18

Flipped and Toppled

The interesting thing about the southern hemisphere is that the seasons are opposite to what we're used to in the north. Spring is fall, winter is summer, and vice versa. So here we were in Pichilemu, Chile, for our Introductory to Biblical Counseling school in September, which was actually the beginning of spring.

Another year had passed, and I was celebrating my 46th birthday. After my traumatic deliverance in DTS and discovering I had misunderstood my life mission, my original dreams and plans for life had definitely been turned on end. My worldview had changed dramatically, and I was seeing things from a new point of view. I was anxious to receive any new counsel, revelation, or insight for my life going forward.

I was keenly aware not to receive man's teaching at face value but instead filter everything through the eyes of the Spirit and God's Word to ensure my new foundation would be based on truth. I was so grateful for the Holy Spirit, who was not only my Comforter but my Teacher, Counselor, and Revealer of wisdom and mysteries. Journal entry September 24, 2006:

"2 Timothy 2, Thank you God for life-for Your Spirit that speaks, even through years of fleshly knowledge. I want

to be set free of bondages of mindsets & be prepared for every good work. I want to ponder & consider, chew & digest everything You speak, so You will give me REAL understanding in everything..."

Pichilemu is a coastal town in Chile that has huge waves and is very popular for surfing. Each base has its own emphasis for their DTS training, and ours was sports. Once again, Larry and I were partnered with our own personal discipler. It was this base's first bilingual counseling school to be offered, so again, we had a large student body. The students in this school were a more mature crowd, with many married couples. There were several other schools going on simultaneously. Due to the lack of space, Larry and I were given a room off-site in a small studio between the school and the beach. It didn't have a good heat source and was flea-ridden, but it was a welcome retreat after our long days of study.

We were thankful for the Internet facilities available at the base so we could stay in contact with family and friends back home. Students were all encouraged to spend personal time with God early prior to breakfast at the base. Larry remained in our room, as I chose to take a short walk to the beach each morning. I had meaningful conversations and was taught life-changing lessons while traveling back and forth from that beautiful place of solace.

Our classroom training began with digging into the wisdom of Proverbs. We were challenged to ask God to reveal false beliefs we'd incorporated into our lives, ask for His truth, and then walk in the light of our new revelation. It was transforming. This began a new discipline for me: reading a Proverb a day. (There is a new one for each day of the month.)

One day, as I was reading from Proverbs 6, it described the six things the Lord hates. This got my attention. The first item up for address popped out in bold lettering: HAUGHTY EYES. God, in His goodness and mercy, informed me that I had haughty eyes. What? Yep, I looked at Larry with haughty eyes. Wow! That wasn't good. I knew that haughtiness comes from pride. I was placing myself above Larry. I was looking down on him. Proverbs 26:12 asks, **"Do you see a man wise in his own eyes? There is more hope for a fool than for him."** I was instantly reminded of when God informed me of His deep love for Larry. I didn't love Larry the way God did. I wanted to.

I asked God where my haughty eyes came from. He told me from my earthly father. Yeah. That resonated as truth. My dad could definitely look at a person with approval or disapproval. Just his glance could make others feel unaccepted and this had alienated him from people, I could do the same. I was faced with my sin. I knew this kept me from experiencing the relationships God wanted for me. Psalms 66:18; **"If I regard wickedness in my heart, The Lord will not hear."** I repented. I asked God to give me the grace to see Larry as He did. I wanted to look at him in a new way, to remove any judgments and recognize him as my equal partner. I knew God heard and answered.

Growing up in the church, I had always believed that God teaches us to forgive and forget. In fact, I was taught that when God forgives us, He throws our sin into the "sea of forgetfulness," never to be remembered again. This, however, is not consistent with scripture. If God truly forgets the past, we'd not have a written account of the majority of our heroes of the faith. The pages of the Bible are flooded with accounts of mistakes, sins, and failures, yet God's love, mercy, and forgiveness override those rebellious acts. Psalms 103:12: **"As far as the east is from the west, so far has He removed our transgressions from us."** They are never to be held against us ever again. His desire is for us to do the same for those who have hurt us. When we choose to forgive from the heart, we still have the memory of our past injustice but no longer feel the pain. Through our free will to forgive, God can turn the ugliest iniquity into a tool of blessing for His children.

Due to living off base, it took more effort to get to know other students, fellowship outside of class, and build relationships. Spring showers brought spring flowers and lots of mud. It was necessary for us to purchase boots, as we often sank into the sticky soil on the way back and forth from class. I started each day with excitement and anticipation, but the dreary days got old quickly for Larry. My discipler questioned me about my personal progress. I shared my new insights learned from Proverbs. I also voiced my disappointment in Larry's constant frustration and my hope for his healing.

This led to sharing our marriage history with her. The behaviors modeled by Larry were narcissistic, and even though I hoped and prayed for a miracle, she offered that my husband might not ever change. I was surprised when my discipler asked why I had stayed in the marriage. She offered that God wouldn't require me to endure the abuse. Yes, I knew the woman was right, but I was thankful that God had clarified my personal mission only a few months prior, His love for my husband, and His trust in me.

My mind wandered to the Old Testament prophet, Hosea. God had asked him to marry a prostitute and father children by her. Later, Gomer, his wife, left Hosea to follow after other lovers. Yes, God was painting a picture of the way Israel had played the harlot after other gods, but Hosea was a real man. He had personal needs and experienced real hurt and betrayal. God gave Hosea the grace and perseverance to go after his wife without any guarantee of healing or restoration. He pursued Gomer to woo her back to himself. What a beautiful picture of God's undying love for us.

The conversation and counsel given by my discipler made

me aware of how important it is for each person to be in the Word and to hear God for themselves. Even with the best intentions, wrong advice can be given even by other believers. No, I was in this for the long haul. I was determined more than ever to follow through with my commitment, for better or for worse.

One of our first classes was on conflict resolution. We were asked to practice our learned skills through a practical hands-on exercise. This infuriated Larry. He was NOT going to participate; in fact, he threatened to quit school and head back home. I informed him that if that was his choice, he needed to leave alone. I was going to finish my school commitment. Journal entry September 29, 2006:

"Thank you God for showing me the revelation of capability. I have been enabling Larry all these years, when he says, "I can't" I should not be the one to jump in and save him. If anyone should be doing the saving, it should be You! I trust You and will obey in this area. I repent for all the many times I got in Your way. I thought I was doing the right thing. I thought I was being kind and the submissive wife. Please break all my deceptions!"

The following morning, I took a different route to my beach. I found myself heading down a hillside bordering a large field surrounded by barbed wire. As I followed the fence line, I realized I was walking parallel to a beautiful white stallion. He'd worn a huge trench in the path along his side of the fence. I was watching my step as I headed down the hill, but he was stomping and snorting as he leaned into the fence line as close as he could. This was causing the barbed wire to dig deeply into his strong, muscular neck. I could see dried blood, as well as new moisture rising to his skin's surface to stain his lovely coat. He was walking faster than me, and as he reached the bottom of the hill, he turned to return on the same path. As he came into my view again, I could see the same wounds on the other side of his neck. Why? He had all of this wonderful, spacious field to run and jump, to have fun and be free! Why would he limit his area and inflict this pain on himself? Then I realized what God was telling me. Larry was being offered freedom, a way of experiencing a smorgasbord of wonders that His Savior had to offer without cost. There were new tools and ways of living at his disposal, but as yet, Larry wasn't willing to trust. He was stuck in his rut. God never violates our free will. He offers the choice. We must decide to receive or reject. I was faced with a new way to pray.

Back in class, we had an interesting lesson on communication. We might believe that others can hear our silence loud and clear, but our actions don't say what we're thinking. The only time in life when a non-spoken message is understood is between a mother and her newborn. Before language is developed, the mother and baby can understand one another through eye contact and touch. The mother can usually tell if the baby is hungry, wet, not feeling well, afraid, tired, or angry. The baby can sense the mother's mood through her touch and body language as well. This response either makes the child feel safe or insecure. Prior to the toddler learning to speak, this communication stops, never to return. So, our spouse can't read our thoughts and, depending on how perceptive they are, may not even notice our body language. Wow! I realized my passive-aggressive behaviors of the past had been a total waste of time.

Over the years, I often responded to Larry by giving him the silent treatment when I was hurt. My train of thought was that he would see and feel my silence, talk to me about the situation, and seek a resolution. It never worked well.

A few days later, I found myself reflecting on the same beach. It was low tide when I saw a small crab that had been washed up on shore. He was on the dry sand, lying on his back, frantically kicking. I watched for some time, hoping he'd be successful in turning himself back over, but to no avail. I looked for a way to help him out and found a big piece of seaweed. I wrapped the tool around the little guy and gently dragged him back into the surf. Feeling proud of myself, I returned to my piece of driftwood and sat down, only to see the waves lift my friend back onto the sand, once again knocking him on his back. The seaweed was close by, so again, I assisted the exhausted crab back into the water. No sooner had I returned to my perch than the small creature was again forced onto the beach as before. This was getting old. I needed to find another approach. I spotted a rock near shore that was surrounded by standing water. If I were to move him into the calm and refreshing pool, he'd be safe until the tide came in. What an ingenious plan. I didn't delay in putting it into action. I then returned to my log and finished my scripture reading without distraction.

The next day, I headed to our meeting place as usual, but as soon as I crested the surrounding hill, I screamed out loud in horror. The entire beach was littered with literally thousands of crabs. They were all dead, and their resting place was their backs! I immediately knew what God was trying to tell me. I couldn't save the world. No matter how good my intentions were, I was wasting my time, spinning my wheels, wearing myself out for naught. I got the message. I repented. Proverbs 19:19: **"A man of great anger will bear the penalty, for if you rescue him, you will only have to do it again."** That day, I finally released Larry totally into the hands of God. I knew that even though I believed my intentions were righteous in trying to make excuses for or "rescuing" Larry, I was operating in a spirit of control.

Attempting to manipulate and control others is the same as witchcraft. Christian or not, any witchcraft is sin. Control is binding another in shackles. They're not free to be themselves or choose on their own. It was hard. I cried out from the depths of my soul. I grieved. It was a true release. What I wasn't aware of at the time was that not only did it loose me from the spirit of control, but there were also powerful, huge chains that dropped off of Larry.

Our next teacher arrived at our school from Uruguay. His class offered a new teaching for me. He invited us to search ourselves to see if there was any area where we had resentment instead of thankfulness. He suggested that thanks should be given even for our most painful experiences and memories. I thought this was heresy! God is good. He doesn't place trauma on us. Sure, we can thank Him for what we've learned through painful experiences, but thank Him for the pain? No! I left class frustrated and in complete disagreement. I did, however, honestly want to have an open heart to receive the truth. I had a lifetime of being wrong with so many of my beliefs. I decided to ask God about it. He directed me to 1 Thessalonians 5:18: **"In everything give thanks; for this is God's will for you in Christ Jesus."** It didn't say for some things or sometimes. Could that mean even in every bad thing, hurt or even abuse? I spent the night meditating on it.

The following day, I returned to class. The teaching resumed. We were again invited to enter into a time of thanksgiving for everything. I was willing to trust God in this. I thanked Him for the most horrific thing I had experienced. I was sincere. I didn't expect what happened next. A joy flooded me. I was truly thankful in a way I had never imagined. God, in His love and all-caring character, knew that without the pain, I could never have experienced the depth of my healing. No, He didn't want me to experience the trauma of being raped by my husband, but He was with me in the pain. My Good Shepherd had always been with me. I thought about Psalm 23. Jesus had truly prepared a table for me, knowing the joy that was set before me after the victory. He was now celebrating with me. I've experienced the reality first-hand of God taking the things that were meant for evil and turning them to good, if we trust and allow Him.

Another important lesson learned in the counseling school was the power of the tongue. It can and is used for blessing or cursing. There are so many times in life where the blessing should've been given, but it's never too late to go back and declare it. Life and death are in the power of the tongue. Proverbs 16:24: **"Pleasant words are a honeycomb, sweet to the soul and healing to the bones."** Not only can I curse through my mouth, but my judgmental and critical thoughts can be just as harmful. It gives permission for bitterness to take root and produce deadly fruit. Hebrews 12:15 warns, **"See to it that no one comes short of the grace of God; that no root of bitterness springing up causes trouble, and by it many become defiled."** I began a new practice of verbally blessing Larry throughout the day and expecting positive results rather than anticipating the worst.

My new experiences, responses, and attitudes were freeing, and I could literally feel the lightness from the load lifted off my body. Jesus was carrying the burden I had claimed as my own for so many years. This changed the atmosphere around me. It also changed my perspective. How could I have been so wrong about so many important things for so long?

God was revealing Himself as the faithful, true Deliverer, the One who sees all, loves, and cares more than I could ever have imagined. He was definitely turning my world upside down, but that was OK. I looked forward to what other surprises might lie ahead.

Our theory phase was drawing to an end. The leaders had arranged for Larry and me to spend our practical outreach phase in Peru. I was filled with anticipation; however, Larry was not doing well. His constant frustration and objection to accepting offered teaching, counsel, or revelation was increasingly manifesting in his body. Instead of walking in freedom, he was experiencing a lot of problems with digestion issues. He found it necessary to take more medications and to be more restrictive in his diet. Thankfully, we were able to buy the medicine we needed more easily in South America. Larry threatened numerous times that he was going to leave school and return to the US, but in the end, he decided to join me in Peru.

**"He who separates himself
Seeks his own desire. He quarrels against
all sound wisdom."
Proverbs 18:1**

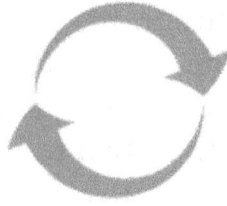

Chapter 19

THE UTTERMOST PARTS OF THE EARTH

We traveled by bus to Peru. As soon as we crossed the border, I was a first-hand witness to the most culturally rich country I had ever experienced. The people were beautiful, their colors vibrant, the music lively, the food exotic, and the hospitality through the roof. I'm not sure if the report was accurate, but I was told the population of the capital city of Lima exceeds that of the entire country of Chile. However, I wouldn't be able to testify to that based on what we saw in Lima. Llama were pulling carts down the streets, peddlers were selling their wares and fruit from their mobile fruit stands, and salesmen were shouting out early in the morning to sell their Sol-gas. It all had a welcoming, small-town, friendly feeling. It was delightful to be immersed in the sights and smells of the culture and to see a people that seemed to remain untouched by Western influence.

We were given a warm send-off from the base with a small budget to last us the full three months. Our team consisted of our leader, Jose from Bolivia, Arlene and Jorge from Brazil, Catalina from Chile, Monique from Brazil, Larry, and me. We committed to work with one main church from Lima. They agreed to house us in apartments, and we put our training into practice by counseling parishioners and leaders in their congregation. The plan was to work in teams. Monique and I were partners. Since Spanish was a 2nd language for us both, we didn't speak too fast and could understand one another fairly well. I had learned a small amount of Portuguese the previous year in my DTS, and she knew pretty much the same amount of English. Catalina, of course, spoke fluent Spanish, and she was teamed up with Arlene. Jorge spoke a fair amount of English, so he was paired with Larry and was prepared to translate. We scheduled appointments in the morning and, in the evenings, offered teaching for those who were interested in attending.

We decided to meet together each morning to discuss issues in the team, appoint the teacher(s) for the evening meeting, and pray together. To kick things off, a humble family from the church invited us to their home in the hills for dinner. It was a very small house, and there wasn't sufficient room for the family to eat with us; besides, they may not even have had enough for themselves, as they continued to bring us plate after plate of food. It was the most amazing hospitality I had ever seen. The kindness and love were overwhelming. We then moved into a small living area filled with resin chairs where the neighbors had been invited to come and hear from the missionaries. It was a wonderful evening that went well into the night.

Later, after arriving back to our room, Larry wasn't well. He reported his diverticulitis was acting up, and he attributed it to all the rice. The following day, he reported to our leader, Jose, that he wasn't feeling well enough to participate in our counseling schedule. Jose filled in to partner with Jorge for the daily appointments. Larry stayed in bed and rested. Our team tailored his meals to avoid roughage, but Larry continued to complain of pain. I offered him his usual treatment of medications, but there was no relief. I would've stayed with him or been more concerned, but Jose advised me not to worry, as he was familiar with the symptoms. He knew it was a spiritual attack, manifesting physically. He'd seen this repeatedly in Bolivia. This gave me peace, as the symptoms grew stronger by the day, and Larry feared he was going to die. God spoke through Psalms 46:10: **"Cease striving and know that I am God."** Time and time again, Larry talked about returning to the States but didn't have the strength or motivation to make the trip. Routinely, on different days, various men from the church came to visit and pray for him.

One night, I sensed a spirit of death over him and spent hours on my knees by his bed, taking authority over the powers of darkness and death that wanted to take Larry out. I prayed for God's mercy to heal and raise him up, but I knew that Larry's free will was the key. I felt impressed to give him a message regarding his choice to accept or reject God's offer of deliverance and freedom. I believed God was offering him a 12-month time frame to accept His grace, but it was a matter of Larry's submission. This message frustrated him, but shortly after, he began to recover. Journal entry February 12, 2007:

> *"Genesis calls me a "helpmeet," but You showed me very clearly today, that my title is a "watchman" Ezekiel 33:6 I didn't know this, but now I do. I take this title seriously. I repent for my unfaithfulness all of these years, for listening to lies from the enemy & believing sometime that it was about me-I know it <u>was</u> about me too, this is how I grew through my mistakes, but now that I have received Your light & truth-I don't want to make the same mistakes or go back. I want to be a faithful watchman."*

Monique and I were amazed each day at how God partnered with us through the counseling sessions. God is balanced as penned in Psalms 89:14: **"Righteousness and justice are the foundation of Your throne; Lovingkindness and truth go before You."** God shows these qualities through

His creation. I'm a mercy and grace type, while Monique ministered through justice and truth. It was awe-inspiring to see the way God seemed only to allow one of us to comprehend at times. Depending on the woman we counseled and her needs, He gave us wisdom to offer the applicable counsel depending on our giftings, while the other one mainly prayed. Occasionally, we both understood and shared things with the women. This happened daily, and it showed how detailed God is, how great and how huge His heart is, and His commitment to personal healing. He loves us so much.

Through our sessions, it was obvious that so many professing Christians are bound by the lies of the enemy. The devil is called the father of lies, and that's what he excels at. Even though I was raised as a child hearing and learning the truth of the Bible and had wonderful examples in my parents and grandparents, I had become deceived myself. I remember the day I took the bait, hook, line, and sinker. As a teenager, I listened to and accepted the enemy's lies, which kept me bound for five years, not even believing there was a God. Even as a follower of God, the devil does all he can to deceive and keep us from the freedom offered by our Heavenly Father. The pride of believing we can live life on our own, acting strong, and thinking we know it all due to our education, degrees, and doctrine is a huge error that leads to downfall. That's why it's so important to stay in the Word of God daily. The Bible is truth. It offers correction and the nourishment needed for our soul and spirit to keep us from deception.

I was very grateful for the opportunity to minister with Monique, as she had years of experience working in deliverance ministry in Brazil. I learned a lot from her about spiritual strongholds and was so blessed to see the women in Peru being set free from bondage. It was the first time for me to work with women in this manner, and I believed and hoped this could be an exciting new avenue of ministry for me in the future.

The time in Peru was quickly nearing an end, so our team met to sum up our experiences. Each of us testified to countless miracles while ministering in the Church through teachings and counseling sessions. Larry shared how thankful he was for the men who came to sit with, encourage, and pray for him while he was bedridden. Immediately, our leader rose up and rebuked him sternly. Jose proclaimed that Larry's wife had been the one to stand in the gap for him daily, praying for his healing and deliverance, and he gave her no acknowledgment. I was taken aback by this bold statement from our leader. I had never expected recognition, but as I respected Jose as an intuitive man of God, I believed the Holy Spirit had led him to speak the words. I was surprised but glad that Larry seemed to accept Jose's admonition and not take offense.

Thankfully, there seemed to be no further health issues as we packed up our little apartment and prepared to head back south to our school base in Chile.

"The works of His hands are truth and justice;
All His precepts are sure.
They are upheld forever and ever;
They are performed in truth and uprightness.
He has sent redemption to His people;
He has ordained His covenant forever;
Holy and awesome is His name."
Psalms 111:7-9

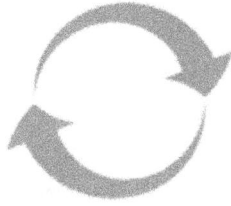

Chapter 20

North, South, East, or West?

We thanked our gracious hosts, exchanged contact information, and said our goodbyes. The land and people of Peru will always hold a special place in our hearts. We returned to our YWAM base in Pichilemu to debrief, receive our graduate diplomas in Biblical Counseling, and prepare to head home. I had the opportunity to check email (which took a long time) at the base. I noticed several messages from the Department of Homeland Security. They were hiring. I knew we would need a sustainable income, so why not? I probably wouldn't qualify, but I decided to apply, regardless.

I was glad to have the opportunity to visit my special beach retreat a few more times. Early one morning, I was taking note as a flock of migrating birds were making their way across the sky. They flew in a V formation, but I noticed after a moment, the lead bird would fall back and another would take his place. This happened several times before they flew out of my view. I heard God speak plainly to me through this picture lesson. "Community is for our health, our protection, and our support. Even creation works as a team. I need to do the same." I was reminded of Proverbs 18:1: **"He who separates himself, seeks his own desire, He quarrels against all sound wisdom."** I made a pledge at that moment to seek out trusted brothers and sisters to share my life with and be accountable to. I knew that in doing so, I would be walking in obedience and safety and find continued healing.

Before flying out of Chile, we were contacted by Sunshine Acres Children's Home, asking if Larry and I would once again cover summer vacations. We agreed, so upon returning to the US, we had a stable place to lay our heads. God is good!

Sometimes, after leaving the mission field, it takes a while to get acclimated back into the familiar surroundings. I had been taught numerous lessons and shown healthy ways of communicating in school. Now, after returning to the US, it was time to put it all into practice. It says in James 1:23-24, **"If anyone is a hearer of the word and not a doer, he is like a man who looks at his natural face in a mirror; for once he has looked at himself and gone away, he has immediately forgotten what kind of person he was."** I was determined not to forget. I never wanted to return to the familiar.

Back in Arizona, I saw a change in Larry. He was withdrawing and spending a lot more time to himself. He rarely accompanied me to church, explaining he was spending his own personal time with God. I realized he was still processing and dealing with many of his own childhood demons, teachings, false beliefs, and religious spirits. He was standing at a fork in the road. He faced choices to change, but change is uncomfortable. My husband could continue in his old patterns or walk in truth. I prayed for him to take the path of life and that this time of introspection would bring him new freedom.

Journal entry March 9, 2007:

"God, You spoke clearly to me. I hear You! I have complete peace to rest in Your words. I know You are a God who gives many chances, but I believe You are just & Your calling to holiness is clear. I WILL wait

the 12 months & trust You. I will also pray that Larry heeds Your voice ... I pray for Your perfect will & take my hands off of trying to control situations the way I see best. I know that You see all. You are the revealer of mysteries. I know what You have planned for me is more than I can imagine. I trust You completely. Only please help me to be faithful to You & not be ashamed or afraid or hide the light You've given to me."

Even after experiencing life-changing freedom through the truth, it's very easy and a temptation to fall back into old responses and patterns. Despite years of personal counseling, mission training, and counseling school, I continued to face the challenges of being sucked into arguments. I was reminded of Dr. Kelly's wisdom to "not get caught up in the dance;" in other words, don't act the way I was expected to, the way I always had. Thanks to the mercy of God, I was choosing to walk in His Spirit. I was a new woman.

I was learning to keep my mouth shut more and to trust. Journal entry March 16, 2007.

"Proverbs 16:23 The heart of the wise instructs his mouth. This is interesting because Your word says that 'From out of the heart the mouth speaks.' The tongue is a deadly poison. So this tells me that when I am truly wise (not wise in my own eyes) my heart will be pure with the right motivation & this wisdom that comes only from God will put great restraint on my tongue to speak the things inspired from the Spirit of God."

James 3:18: **"The seed whose fruit is righteousness is sown in peace by those who make peace."**

I waded through many years of hoping, praying, and striving for peace. I truly believed it was my job to help Larry see the light. I thought that if I could only see the dreams fulfilled of my husband and I serving together on the mission field, I would be satisfied. I would have finally arrived at my—our—lifelong destination. Now, after attending mission school and living a couple of years in foreign countries, I wondered if I had been off-track. God clearly showed me my primary purpose and mission was to show His love to my husband, but I just knew there was more in store. I was asking for direction and which way to turn.

It seems that nearly every day, I put into practice new ways of responding and was tested to see God's provisions for myself. Journal entry March 23, 2007:

> *"Larry's relationship with God must come from his own heart and not what I hope for him. In this time of waiting, it's hard for me. I am tempted to speak, but I need to take my hands off & instead check my own heart & seek God's will & personal word for my life. It is sad & hard not to see my hopes realized for us together, but I need to obey & move on. I commit all my mind, heart, soul, will & emotions to this my God."*

Remembering the lesson of the birds, I was actively praying for and looking for my accountability team, but not yet having a confirmation of who that was, I continued to struggle, seemingly alone. Journal entry; March 28, 2007:

> *"God, here I am, and nothing has changed. Larry is not sorry, at least his words, attitude, body language or actions don't show it. He just wants to move on like all his life & ignore there is a problem. Any problem is mine. There is no conflict resolution. I am to the point of giving up. PLEASE, take my hands totally off. Deal with it in Your perfect, just way. I am helpless. That is the way I always should have looked at it though, I know I've never been in control, even though I've tried. Please forgive me. I trust You."*

I wish I would have understood and trusted those many

years back the wisdom offered in Isaiah 40:28-31: **"Have you not known? Have you not heard? The everlasting God, the Lord, The Creator of the ends of the earth, neither faints nor is weary. His understanding is unsearchable. He gives power to the weak, and to those who have no might, He increases strength. Even the youths shall faint and be weary, and the young men shall utterly fall, but those who wait on the Lord shall renew their strength; they shall mount up with wings like eagles, they shall run and not be weary, they shall walk and not faint."** I recognized that when I was tempted to be impatient and stressed, I wasn't trusting. I wanted to trust and experience true rest.

The object lesson of the beach crabs came to mind often, and with God's help, I no longer attempted to "help Larry out" with his decision-making. As I respected his free choice and removed my hands of control, I noticed Larry was also loosening his grip on me and allowing me to pursue my personal interests without becoming as frustrated. I was able to sense a shift in the spiritual atmosphere and experience personal freedom I had never felt since marrying.

Thankfully, I was starting to recognize the spirit of strife sooner and responding in new ways. Proverbs 26:20-21: **"For lack of wood the fire goes out, and where there is no whisper, contention quiets down, Like charcoal to hot embers and wood to fire, So is a contentious man to kindle strife."** Journal entry, January 28, 2008:

"Well, here I am again-it seems that my desperation drives me to the place of reflection & introspection. Once again I am reminded of the path I'm on, Your voice of direction & kind nudge. I can see the spots where I've taken 5 steps back into the area of comfort. Change is uncomfortable, hard & it hurts. Especially for me since I like peace & comfort. I take Your trust in

me very seriously, so I'll move forward in obedience
even though others may judge, misunderstand & even
criticize. What You think is the most important."

Looking back, I could see that there were months of journaling on the subject. As soon as I received the reminders, I was given the chance to put new choices into life practice. Proverbs 22:10: **"Drive out the scoffer, and contention will go out, even strife and dishonor will cease**." Proverbs 17:14: **"The beginning of strife is like letting out water, so abandon the quarrel before it breaks out."**

When I saw the signs of aggression, I was changing my response. If the atmosphere became uncomfortable, I was learning to remove myself from the stressful situation by going for a walk or leaving the house. This helped to prevent me from getting caught up in arguments or being tempted to fight back in the flesh. I'm proof that no one is ever too old to change. God was helping me to establish and practice safe boundaries.

But change does not automatically make things easy. On February 8, 2008, I penned my battle:

"It's hard for strife to survive alone, isn't it? It is one of
the things You HATE, in fact it is an abomination to You.
If You feel so strongly about it, why do I stick around??
This is an amazing revelation. I'm not supposed to
participate with it! It is a spirit that traps everyone in its
path. Staying away from strife is an attitude of the heart
& act of the will. (desire & obedience) Psalm 31:20 You
promise to shelter me when I can't physically remove
myself. Prov 28:25 Pride, arrogance causes strife & also
allows or participates in it. That's why I MUST leave.
Rom 13:13 These are all sins we participate in. (free
will) James 3:16 Strife brings confusion. Gal 5:20 It's
one of the deeds of the flesh that God instructs us to
NOT participate with. I am obeying + being free from

the binding power of the enemy when I walk away. The devil would lie & say I am being arrogant, proud, self-righteous when I leave, but with the right attitude of heart, I am 100% in obedience & in the plans of God to do so. Please help me God to walk out this revelation in a new way. Please give me victory in this area, as well as Larry & our kids. Set Larry free from this awful bondage of strife. Help him to walk in freedom as he submits his will to Yours, please. Thank You!"

After we all settled into our living quarters and returned to the relief houseparent role, I received a follow-up email from Homeland Security. They accepted my application and requested information for background checks. I was surprised but had peace to continue the process. Step by step, things moved ahead, and amazingly, I was approved each step of the way.

As I continued to pray and ask for God to reveal the dark areas in my own life, I felt encouragement and victory. I was beginning to understand, in a new way, the authority of Jesus and how He desired me to appropriate that daily. Journal entry February 27, 2008:

"I understand & desire that my life can be an extension of Your peace to others. When my feet are dressed with Your peace-when I am experiencing it in my life personally, just my walk into an area of chaos or strife-the presence of God through me, can cut through that spirit & bring hope & victory. That is my prayer. I am in Your army to bring REAL peace, not compromising or pacifying, but healing face-to-face truth from You, that sets the captive free."

I recalled my frustration prior to our Arizona move. I had felt as if I was trapped in that perpetual roundabout of chaos, and there was no way out. God had challenged me that day to trust Him, and He proved Himself faithful each step of the way. I was becoming keenly aware that the battlefield began in my mind. The choice of how to respond, either in the flesh or the spirit, starts there. The battle could be won from the get-go if I insisted and commanded my thoughts to submit to God. 2 Corinthians 10:5 says, **"We are destroying speculations and every lofty thing raised up against the knowledge of God, and we are taking every thought captive to the obedience of Christ."**

Larry didn't share many of his personal thoughts and decisions during those months of adjustment, but I knew he was choosing life. I was glad for him and praised God for His patience and faithfulness. It couldn't be seen with the naked eye, but I could sense something was changing inside Larry, and it was good.

In June, I received confirmation that I was officially hired for a TSA position to work at an airport. I was sent a list of openings and given the option to pick a location. With Larry's input, we narrowed the choices down to Yakima or Wenatchee in Washington State or Saipan Island in the South Pacific (Still dreaming of exotic places for mission work). I was called back and offered the position at YKM, the airport in Yakima, Washington, to begin on October 3, 2008.

We began looking for housing. Now and then, my new supervisor would call to check up on me and ask about my moving progress. He would often ask questions to see how much I knew about the area. Yakima was known for gang violence, drugs, and a very large Hispanic population. "Was I really sure I wanted to move there?" I told him none of that concerned me. It was mid-September. We gave notice of our move to SACH. We found a duplex to rent in Yakima, submitted our security deposit and 1st and last month's rent, and signed a one-year lease. Larry's brother and family had committed to come to Arizona to help us with our move. Everything was arranged.

One night, two weeks prior to the move, I had a very vivid dream. I dreamed I lost my job and was crying hysterically. It was so real; I woke myself up crying. As I sat up in bed, I heard God ask me, "Haven't I always taken care of you?"

"Yes," was my response. "You always have."

I calmly laid back down and returned to sleep. The next morning, I received a phone call from my new supervisor. Due to the economic downsizing, my job in Yakima was cut. He could offer me 24 hours a week in Spokane (3 1/2 hours away), but otherwise, I didn't have a job. I wasn't shocked. I wasn't worried. God had prepared me. I thanked my supervisor but declined his offer. We were prepared to move to Yakima.

"Be on the alert, stand firm in the faith,
act like men, be strong.
Let all that you do be done in love."
1 Corinthians 16:13-14

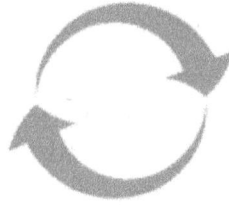

Chapter 21

A Mission in My Backyard

It was the fall of 2008 and in the heart of the economic downturn when I turned 48. Larry's brother and wife came to Arizona to assist us in loading up the U-Haul and to help drive the vehicles northwest for the 2 1/2-day journey. Both Larry and I had resigned from our positions at Sunshine Acres to move to a new town, sight unseen, with no jobs.

We were thankful to be met by some new friends in Yakima who helped us unload our belongings into our three-bedroom rental. We were all praying for direction and provision. The first thing I set about to do was to familiarize myself with the community. I visited the local Union Gospel Mission, met with the director of another homeless outreach, visited a local youth center, and researched various ministries in the area. I knew God had specifically moved us to Yakima, but I still didn't know why.

Even though I didn't have a clue what lay ahead, I had an unexplainable excitement and anticipation stirring inside of me. We set out to find a church right away. Since we had enjoyed the informal setting of our Saturday night service in Arizona, we searched for Saturday options for Christian fellowship in Yakima. This led us to our new church home. Larry opted to enjoy his private worship at home, mostly. I was thankful while recognizing my own self-growth. Years before, I would've tried to pressure Larry to attend with me for "his own good." I could see that letting go of my own control was setting Larry free to be himself, and he was making great choices with his freedom. I found it interesting that the more I trusted him in God's hands, the less Larry tried to control me. He continued taking medication for impulsive behaviors but would still experience frequent outbursts of anger.

Remembering God's picture lesson of the birds, I prayed for wisdom for whom to share my personal story. God highlighted our new pastor and his wife, as well as a church elder and his spouse. We met one afternoon at a Chinese restaurant, where I gave my testimony and marriage history and voiced my desire to be accountable to and come under Christian leadership for counsel. We exchanged cell phone numbers, and my new prayer partners committed to pray whenever the need arose. The following week, I found it necessary to text my friends during an explosive and abusive episode. We immediately agreed together in prayer, and I was excited to see how quickly God answered. You may not believe this, but I only found it necessary to contact them this one time. My steps of obedience, trusting, and becoming vulnerable to others changed the environment. It broke chains in the spiritual realm, and I felt safe from that day forward. Praise God!

Within a month of moving, I was hired as a case manager, working night shifts at a lockdown crisis center for runaway youth. As you can imagine, many of the kids were full of rebellion, but I was able to have conversations with and build relationships with a few of them. One young man stood out in particular. Samuel would often run away with his girlfriend to get away from the eyes of authority. He had a problem with rules, policies, and procedures but also exhibited a fun-loving attitude. He enjoyed debating and participating in serious talk. As he found himself at our facility on a regular basis, it wasn't long before trust was built between us, and we often engaged in thought-provoking discussions.

Not long after, I was asked by the pastor of our new church to head up a local mission and outreach ministry, which I was delighted to do. I had a vision to partner with other local churches to work together rather than starting lots of new programs. La Casa Hogar was one of the organizations we partnered with. They assisted with homeless and emergency services for those experiencing economic crises. I began volunteering there and loved it. It wasn't long before I was offered a job to work there as a case manager. I agreed, and since Larry still hadn't found work, I continued working my night shift with the crisis youth.

After our move, my parents began a new tradition by driving four hours northeast and visiting us yearly to celebrate the New Year and Dad's birthday. It was also an excuse to check up on us and see what was happening in our neck of the woods in Central Washington. My dad enjoyed going with me on the weekend to serve meals to the homeless while my mom remained back at the house for bonding time with Larry.

Dad had been volunteering for years by ministering to the shut-ins at three different senior centers weekly and had finally received his ordination to become an official chaplain. I could see now, more than ever, how Christian service played such an important role in his mind for success. My dad had always encouraged our family to be diligent in serving. If others didn't share his passion for ministry, he could come across as judgmental, and people would feel alienated by him. I began to pray for my dad to receive new revelation for his own freedom from works and for him to have the ability as a leader to be the example for setting all of our family free.

I felt as if my kaleidoscope was coming into focus. All my adult life, I had looked for and had been searching for my place in ministry. I had traveled to faraway countries praying for a place to settle, but here in Yakima, I felt a sense of purpose I had never experienced before. I often spoke more Spanish than English at work. I was working right in the midst of the broken, hurting, and needy homeless population. It was as if I were born, raised, and trained for a lifetime to work in the heart of Yakima. Furthermore, I knew I would have detested airport security. I shared in a hearty belly laugh with Father God, as He had amazingly orchestrated the job, and TSA was the route to move me here. Proverbs 5:21 says, **"The ways of a man are before the eyes of the Lord, and He watches all his paths."**

One day, I purchased a book for my sister for her upcoming birthday. I knew I could mail the package at a reduced book rate. While paying the postage, I informed the postmaster that I would like to purchase the stamp accordingly. He asked if the package contained any correspondence, to which I answered, "No." While preparing to leave and return to my car, I was confronted with my answer. "You said there was no correspondence, but you included a card." Yes, I had thought of that when asked but had dismissed that still small voice. I returned to the counter to speak with the same customer service representative and confessed that the package contained a handwritten card. The extra postage was added to the package, and I left with a clear conscience. Journal entry July 8, 2009:

"Do not despise small beginnings. If I'm faithful with the small things, I can be trusted with the big. I can't imagine what is ahead. Zech 4:10"

I'm so thankful for the Holy Spirit's gentle correction to light our path and keep us headed in the right direction.

In September 2009, Larry was hired to stock the new Wal-Mart opening up down the road. After completing the process, he was offered the position of Photo-Tech. As photography was one of his greatest interests, this was a great fit for him. Even though he would come home and complain about the job daily, it was obvious that he was challenged by and enjoyed the work.

When Larry began working, I gave up my night position and devoted extra time to volunteering in the community. I was able to get to know the homeless population in a more intimate way on weekends as I served sandwiches with friends. Several individuals who lived on the street came to receive their US mail at our outreach office, and I knew a lot of their personal stories.

One day, while I was driving through town, I saw a man holding a sign on the street corner asking for money. I knew him and was aware that he received food and Social Security benefits. Immediately, I felt judgments begin to rise up in my heart. God sternly admonished me, "Watch out for those haughty eyes!" At once, I repented and thanked God from the bottom of my heart, acknowledging that it was only by His grace that I wasn't standing in the same spot as this man. Proverbs 30:12-13 says, **"There is a kind who is pure in his own eyes, yet is not washed from his filthiness. There is a kind-oh how lofty are his eyes! and his eyelids are raised in arrogance."**

If I truly wanted to be effective in this place of ministry, I needed to look at others through the eyes of our Father. I thanked God for the gentle reminder. His love is SO great! Journal entry Oct 27, 2009:

> *"God, I trust You when You said, 'I can't imagine what You have planned for me!' I still am not sure what this means, but I believe You. You are awesomely good! Because of this, I know what You have planned is good, whether here or with You. I believe what You have planned for Larry & each of my children is equally good, righteous, just & fits their mold perfectly!"*

As we neared the year's end, I reflected on God's amazing care and direction in our lives. I knew I had found a true mission field right in the heart of Yakima. I had never expected to be in a place of such peace and contentment. I was finally good with letting go of life's steering wheel and to fully trust in His leading.

**"Let's consider how to stimulate one another
to love and good deeds,
not forsaking our own assembling together,
as is the habit of some,
but encouraging one another;
and all the more as you see
the day drawing near."
Hebrews 10:24-25**

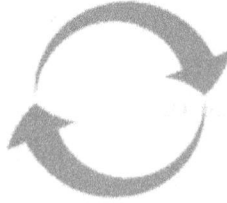

Chapter 22

THE GRASS WITHERS, THE FLOWER FADES

The New Year of 2010 found my daughter asking me for wedding advice. She had met the man of her dreams through her own involvement with mission training. I was delighted to be involved and attend the international wedding with her brother, Lucas. I was excited and extremely blessed to have another son in the family.

I returned home to Yakima safe and sound and was excited to share all the wedding details with Larry, who had stayed behind. He was anxiously looking forward to putting a wedding album together with all the photos. Lucas also made plans to visit us after leaving the wedding; however, his flight was delayed for several weeks due to an unexpected volcano. I sure was glad I made it home before the eruption.

Settling back into the swing of things at work, it was hard to concentrate at times, with my mind and part of my heart 1/2 the world away. After the volcano calmed down, Lucas arrived to share his stories and adventures of international travel. It was fun to discuss our mutual wedding experiences. Although I was not certain, I think Larry may have felt left out a bit. I enjoyed morning walks and conversations with Lucas. When discussing my approval of and excitement about having a son-in-law in the family, he advised me to revel in the enjoyment, as he would never marry. My response was that I had prayed for his mate since he was a baby, and I had faith. He stated that he wished he could share my optimism, but it was impossible as he could never find a person who would be compatible with his lifestyle.

The time went by quickly, and Larry and I were sad to see Lucas leave so soon to return to his teaching job in Indonesia. I was aware of how fast my life was passing and began meditating on the relativity of time. Journal entry June 27, 2010:

> *"God, You don't live in time, we do. You are eternal-we are too, but in this life You work in time for us-mankind. Joseph was placed in time for a purpose. Eccl 3:1 There is a time appointed for everything under heaven. Eccl 8:6-7 There are proper times-none of us know. Genesis 18:14 There is the fullness of time. Eph 1:10 Signs of the times, due time and end time."*

It is amazing how quickly time flies. According to James 4:14, **"Yet you do not know what your life will be like tomorrow. For you are just a vapor that appears for a little while, and then vanishes away."** I was becoming increasingly aware of how fast time slips away. More than ever, I wanted my life to count.

Through my mission contacts at church and my given responsibility at work as a representative for our agency in the Association of Churches in Yakima County, I was glad to meet many of the pastors and become acquainted with various ministries in town. Samuel, the young man I had met while working with runaway youth, started coming to our church and was mentored by one of the men there. He seemed to be doing well. I also worked with him through my homeless outreach job to help and encourage him.

I celebrated my 50th birthday in September with neither

of my children in the country. A year later, Larry and I were so excited to welcome our kids to the Emerald City of Seattle on Mother's Day, 2011.

Also, 2011 brought about a change in my job. A local community health clinic took over our agency's homeless outreach and emergency services. A co-worker and I were both assimilated into the company, but not without a stern warning from the company's CEO regarding proselytizing. She knew me from previous dealings in the community and knew I was a Christian.

Larry had sought out and found a new mental health provider in Yakima who was monitoring his health as well as the efficiency of his medications. Larry invited me to accompany him to one of his appointments. He was taking his medication as prescribed while working his job but not taking it regularly on his days off. The doctor asked my opinion regarding Larry's routine. I noted the meds helped him with his impulsiveness and anger, but Larry didn't realize the importance of taking them for stability at home and to help with interpersonal relationships. After discussing the pros and cons, Larry agreed his family was a priority and decided to change his habits and attempt to take his medications daily. This helped immensely, made our times together more enjoyable, and helped Larry feel better about himself. Even though I definitely realized the benefits of the medications, I still believed that God desired to heal Larry and continued to trust in prayer for that.

Around this time, I found a spot on my skin that I believed needed attention, and I scheduled an appointment with the dermatologist. The doctor told me the spot in question was not a concern, but I had an area in the middle of my face that needed to be tested. His keen eye proved to be right, as it was cancerous. The surgery would be exploratory, and since it was right in the middle of my cheek, they would not cut in deeper than necessary. In the end, I needed to return three times under the knife to get all the surrounding cancer cells removed. The hole ended up being the size of a quarter but 3x the thickness. I'm thankful the doctor was also a skillful plastic surgeon who was able to stretch my skin to pull the scar down as far as my smile line.

Larry was extremely concerned during the whole cancer scare. He couldn't articulate the change in his way of thinking towards me, but something extraordinary had happened inside. Responses were different. Larry was more appreciative. I witnessed him becoming kinder, less critical, and more loving. He extended grace when I didn't finish my projects in a timely manner. He didn't push me to get things done like he'd done in the past and was willing to help out more with household chores. I was delighted to see the way that Larry was beginning to question me about my feelings and opinions more often. He even began to ask my advice on purchases. The cool thing is that it didn't just last during my recovery time. I was so thankful for what was happening. It was a real-life miracle.

There were times I had nearly given up on believing in real change in my marriage. I don't know if the visual scar across the left side of my face was a constant reminder of my fragility, but nonetheless, something inside Larry's heart was being transformed for good. One day, he shared with me a new revelation. He had recently been reading Matthew 13, which described a merchant seeking fine pearls. After finding one of great value, he went and sold everything he had to buy it. Larry confided that, in a moment, he realized I was that pearl. In the days following, I witnessed my husband becoming a softer, more caring man. I was once again reminded to give thanks from my heart for everything, the good and the bad.

Larry began to talk about retirement and seemed to be doing better with his out-of-control spending; however, he found it difficult to make the due dates on two of his credit cards. He promised to cut them up if I helped him with the payments. In hopes of finally clearing up our debt for good, I agreed. I did make it clear to him that this was the last time I would pay toward his credit debt. Larry agreed, and we decided together that when all credit cards were paid in full, he could finally retire from all outside employment.

After successfully coming out on the other end of our family health concerns, Larry and I committed to never again take each other for granted. There was a new awareness that our lives were out of our own hands and every individual has the right to be valued, appreciated, celebrated, and treated with respect, love, and care. Life is short. Youthful beauty fades. True beauty comes from the heart of Father God. It is revealed in our new character and manifests through humility and a willingness to grow.

**"Blessed be the God and Father
of our Lord Jesus Christ,
The Father of mercies and God of all comfort,
Who comforts us in all our affliction
So that we will be able to comfort those who are
in any affliction
With the comfort with which we ourselves are
comforted by God."
2 Corinthians 1:3-4**

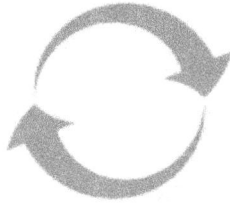

Chapter 23

Expanding our Territory

Larry was beginning to attend church more regularly with me. We felt led to become a part of another church fellowship in Yakima. Our new church was a younger crowd, but we loved our pastor, who was real and transparent with a genuine heart for the lost. Rather than people-pleasing, obeying God was his main priority. I was delighted that Larry was finally excited to accompany me to church.

Our family did not feel complete, however, with Lucas on the other side of the planet. He had a brilliant idea to invite us to share a vacation with him in Indonesia. We arranged to meet him in Bali, and Lucas planned the entire agenda. I was excited to visit a new country. There is a promise in the Bible in Deuteronomy 11:24 that says, **"Every place on which the sole of your foot treads shall be yours..."** In March 2013, we put footsteps into action, and what a time we had. We loved the culture and people. Even though they are bound by the false religion of Hinduism, God loves the people of Bali. We visited coffee plantations, beaches, and temples and enjoyed a wonderful visit with staff at a local YWAM base. It would've been a perfect trip if I had not crashed a moped, breaking my arm and cracking my ribs. I will think twice before ever renting a moped again in a foreign country. In the end, I believe my feet made a difference in that tropical foreign land, even while walking the halls of a strange hospital while high on painkillers!

Back at home, I was serving on the prayer team at church, and often, I would arrive early on Sunday to spend time in the room set aside for prayer before service. Usually, there would be several people there, but one winter morning, the room was bare, probably because of the heavy snowfall outside. I was looking out the window while talking to God and wondering about the beauty of winter. The snow was falling gracefully and landing on an old oak tree in front of me. My curiosity prompted the question, "God, I've heard that every snowflake is unique, like a fingerprint. Do you fashion each one, or does it happen naturally through physics or such?" Immediately, I saw two snowflakes forcibly launched from the treetop at a steep incline. It reminded me of Larry and Lucas back in the day when they raced their pinewood derby cars. Each snowflake was trying to outrun the other until they reached their final destination on the ground. In an instant, everything returned to calm as before. God had made His answer clear. I was amazed that day at His picture story and continue to be in awe of His personal demonstrations of love, detail, and care.

After being a part of the counseling team in Peru, I realized the huge need and God's desire for His children to walk in freedom. Ever since moving to Yakima, I kept my eyes out, looking for ways to become a part of some type of deliverance ministry. When I heard of SOZO, I did some research and sought out training to become involved. With the blessing of our pastor, I went through the required training to become part of a ministry team in the area. I had never been more blessed or excited to be involved with anything in my life. Every time we ministered to those truly seeking God's healing, we saw people transformed and miracles happen right before our eyes.

For years, I prayed to have a close friend with whom I

could confide and be vulnerable and real. When Susie and I met, we just clicked. She was eleven years older than me, but the two of us could spend time together, and before you knew it, hours would pass. She also struggled for many years with mental illness and was able to give me real insight into relating to Larry. She explained that whenever Larry blew up, it was because he was afraid, and I shouldn't take it personally. Every time we were together, I returned home and seemed to be more understanding of Larry's responses. He actually liked me spending time with Susie. I seemed to be an encouragement to her, too. We'd talk like magpies, and when we were apart, we'd pray for one another and our respective families. We found ourselves growing mutually each time we met.

I've always had a burden and love for the people of Haiti. After speaking with our pastor and receiving the blessing from my husband, I led a team from our church to go there in July 2014.

We had fun getting to know one another while participating in various fundraising projects. The plan was to meet up with a mission team in Miami, fly to Port-au-Prince, and, with the help of a security guard, minister in remote areas of the country. Each one of us was challenged during the trip to share our personal stories and to offer hope to individuals bound by witchcraft. We had numerous opportunities to speak to large crowds, encouraging them to become a part of a local, Bible-believing community. We saw miracles of deliverance happen before our eyes as we participated in outdoor crusades. All of us left Haiti with new friends and enlarged hearts for the beautiful people.

Lucas returned to Yakima in 2014. He had walked across entire countries in Asia but now decided he wanted to do the same in the USA. He became acquainted with a wonderful dog, Buddy, whom Lucas trained to walk without a leash and stay and come upon command. The two of them crossed the country on foot, and a bond was formed between them that is rare to find. Buddy was in an accident in Montana, which left him with three legs, but his determination didn't stop him from completing the goal of reaching the East Coast in just over 6 months. Lucas blogged the entire trip. It can be found on the web at https://walking-eastward.blogspot.com/. After the completion of his walk, Lucas trained for and obtained his CDL license and began trucking long-haul across the country with Buddy by his side.

In April 2016, we were successful in surprising my parents with a 75th birthday celebration for them both in Tennessee. It wasn't an easy task for my brothers and sisters, my mom's sister, and our kids to make the trip and secretly arrive ahead of time to prepare the large condo for their arrival. My mom and dad thoroughly enjoyed our time together as we did a lot of hiking, explored the Smoky Mountains, and, to finish off the trip, visited the Creation Museum, of which my dad was a loyal financial supporter and founder.

In the spring of 2017, Lucas once again invited Larry and me to accompany him on an adventure to Mongolia. We hoped to experience the culture and stay with the hospitable nomadic families of the step (pasture land of Mongolia) in their yurts. How could we turn that opportunity down? It was freezing cold, but that didn't stop us from helping to herd goats, riding camels in the snow, and mounting the hardy Mongolian horse. I made personal bracelets for the women with different colored stones to share the gospel. It was interesting that the colors were nearly identical to those of their Buddhist prayer flags. Our translator, Boggie, became so familiar with the gospel story that she was nearly able to share it on her own by the end of our time together. I pray the bracelets will continue to bear fruit even years later. Once again, we were grateful to participate in the trip of a lifetime.

Larry and I returned home to work and Lucas to trucking

that March, which he continued until Buddy's untimely death that summer. Lucas was heartbroken, and seeing his hurt, I shared in the brokenness. Together, Lucas and I traveled with Buddy to Central Oregon to lay his body to rest. He was buried near the spot where his childhood dog, Sandy, was laid more than 20 years prior on our family property. God created Buddy as Lucas' special, loyal companion. He was a precious gift who could never be replaced.

After settling back into the flow of daily activities, I took time to reflect and acknowledge that God had miraculously led Larry and me to Yakima. I realized that since we were married, this was the longest period the two of us had ever lived in the same city and place. There was a sense of being home. Since learning to trust Larry in God's care, I was truly experiencing peace and rest. We were enjoying family, finally building relationships, and making memories. I recognized that while we were honoring God's priorities, we were still making an impact on other nations. God was warming both my mission and my mother's heart.

**"Taste and see that the Lord is good;
How blessed is the man who takes refuge in Him!"
Psalm 34:8**

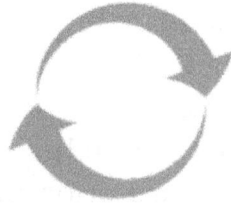

Chapter 24

A TIME FOR MIRACLES

My mom had always had a dream of taking a family cruise. On the other hand, it was the last thing in the world on my dad's bucket list. My father believed in hard work and, in his mind, cruises were a waste of time and money and a place to be pampered. In July 2017, we kids again gifted them with a trip. It was an Alaskan cruise, and against his better judgment, my dad agreed to go. My mom was thrilled to spend the time with her kids and grandkids and to enjoy some pampering herself.

Since my revelation of "haughty eyes," I had been praying for my dad to have his own revelation and be set free for himself. Journal entry July 2, 2017:

"Well, at this point I have not seen the evidence, but Heb 11 says, 'Faith is the substance of things hoped for...' I hope & trust for the new things today. Is this the environment for you to reveal new things of life to Dad? I am asking, claiming & believing for those strong chains of pride & false belief systems to be broken & torn down to the foundation. For new-healthy foundational stones to be laid down-for joy & compassional love & acceptance & for the haughty eyes to be gone- to see from Your loving, forgiving eyes."

I continued writing July 5, 2017:

"I pray & believe that Dad will experience Your joy & abundant life. He is so important to our family & has influence in so many other lives. The enemy does not want him to live life the way You desire, nor be able to share that with others. I look back on so many years of my life & all I can say is 'Thank You from the bottom of my heart.' I love You & would not change any hardship or trial for the joy I am living in You!"

Despite my dad's feelings, I believe he enjoyed the trip, and we were thankful for all the precious memories created.

In January 2018, I was reunited with Samuel. He had served some time in prison, was released, and then relapsed on drugs. This led to him attempting to end his own life. He ended up in a mental hospital, where God reminded him of His love. Samuel came to my job asking for job readiness assistance, and as I was working in that capacity, I was thankful for the opportunity to collaborate with him. He was self-motivated to get his GED, and with my help, he completed his training with honors and then proceeded to work on his driver's test and get his license. His exemplary achievements qualified him to work as an intern for our community health clinic. He was hired and did a fantastic job. He also started serving in a local church using his talents in IT and video. He loved being a part of the ministry, built lots of healthy relationships, and was appreciated. Soon after, he met a wonderful Christian woman and fell in love.

That summer, unbeknownst to Larry and me, Lucas had been communicating with and getting to know a woman online at the suggestion of his sister. Though unknown at the beginning, she and Lucas had mutual friends in common. The young woman, Heather, was also a missionary who had ministered overseas for years. She was now in the USA while on a sabbatical and staying with her parents in Colorado.

I had the opportunity to join in on a 2 1/2-week mission trip to Uganda. Larry not only was allowing me to go, but at this point, I felt I had his full support and encouragement for me to be involved in ministry. Our small team of four was participating in fundraising projects and accepting donations. My parents wanted to be involved and had given a large financial gift to help support the trip. We loaded numerous suitcases with items to bless the local people and orphans, mostly refugees from South Sudan. We were to team up with a YWAM mission family from the area, who were very experienced in working with refugees.

We left in mid-August and flew into the Kampala Entebbe Airport in the south of Uganda. I stood in awe at the beauty of the landscape and people as penned in my Journal entry on August 31, 2018:

".. The way You care for every detail of creation, shows Your thought & intent that never leaves out a detail. Every species provided for-never lacking-How could I think You might forget about what lies ahead for me?"

We traveled to the northwest corner of the country by bus to Arua, where we ministered to children at the YWAM base and refugees in the community. We then traveled east to a children's orphanage near the South Sudan border. We were the first visitors ever to arrive there. They were so excited to see us. These were all children who were orphaned by the war in S. Sudan.

While visiting the orphanage, I was invited to speak to the women who cared for the children. I prayed about the topic and felt I should share my personal story of abuse and betrayal in my marriage. I talked about the wounding, the need for forgiveness, and the hope of God's healing. As we sat in the shade of the trees next to the community well, I noticed that as I was willing to be vulnerable and share my heart, women began to weep. So many of them had suffered unspeakable abuse, not only from husbands but during war and at the hands of border patrols. As I had the opportunity to pray with the women, I was told how surprised they were to learn that they could relate to a Christian white woman from America who had overcome pain. I was humbled and thankful that I could be used as a vessel for several women to be set free and delivered that day.

Our hearts were so touched by the children. Later, after returning and sharing our stories, our home church in Yakima adopted the same orphanage to continue assisting with expanding wells, gardening and agriculture, and building projects to add safe sleeping quarters.

We returned to Arua to minister in a prison. We worshipped in the rain while prisoners played with all their hearts on their homemade instruments. We were invited to visit with a pastor's family who had a tiny shack. We were greeted with, "You are most welcome." They brought out a piece of plywood and mounted it on a stump outside. To beautify it, they covered it with a piece of fabric. They gave us all a plastic resin chair (they are everywhere, provided by the UN) to sit on. They then brought around a pitcher of water to wash our hands. At this point, it was difficult to hold back the tears. They provided us with their best of peanuts and soda pop. They were on the edge of their seats, so hungry to hear the message from the American missionaries. We were definitely the ones who were ministered to and blessed the most!

That night, I received a message from Larry. My dad had suffered a massive stroke and was found in bed unresponsive. He was in a coma. The doctors didn't think Dad would make it. I needed to get back quickly. But it would be a full day's journey by bus to the airport, and it wouldn't be safe for me to travel alone. I decided to wait and return as planned with our team. That night, I prayed harder than ever.

I cried out to God to spare my dad. Even though I knew

my father was saved and would go to heaven, I told God he wasn't ready, and I begged Him to please not let him go until he was really free. I didn't sleep much that night. Thankfully, Larry was able to contact me with updates.

My brother is a nurse and was by my father's side constantly, declaring he'd live and not die. Our son Lucas' lady friend, Heather, had previously agreed to fly into Portland, Oregon, to meet him for the first time in person. He picked her up at the airport, and they went straight to the hospital to see his grandpa. I was informed that Lucas prayed in the hospital room in Hindi while Heather prayed in another tongue. According to those present in the room, during those prayers, my dad responded for the first time by squeezing their hand.

Larry knew how close I was to my dad. He was waiting at the arrival gate of Seattle Airport to whisk me immediately to the hospital. My dad was now conscious, but due to his massive stroke, he was full of tubes, paralyzed on his right side, unable to eat or relieve his bladder or bowels, and unable to speak. In his compassion, Larry had purchased a gold bracelet for me, engraved with the words, "Family is Everything." It was precious and touched my heart.

Since my brother and mom had been with him non-stop for more than a week, I volunteered to spend the night at the hospital. Larry was very understanding of my feelings. My dad slept a lot, but when he was awake, he was interested in hearing about the mission trip and looking at pictures. He was a proud man, and his limitations caused him to break down often, and I would embrace him as we cried together. This was the beginning of coming once a month to spend a weekend with him and give my mom a break. Journal Entry September 14, 2018:

"You have given the choices set before me each day- the blessings or the curse. Everything You want for me

is good. I am the one who brings hardships, delays, disappointments on myself when I choose my own way. I want to choose life & trust You completely with Dad & all he is going through. Help me to be an instrument of love & healing to him & others in the family. 11 Thessalonians 1:11-12 so all God's desires & purposes will be fulfilled in Dad & all our family."

I learned that after Lucas left the hospital, he went to visit his great-grandmother to introduce Heather. They then traveled to the beach to spend time getting acquainted in person. Larry and I learned all these details secondhand from family members who felt privileged to meet this mystery woman. On speaking to my grandma on the phone, I knew she believed that Heather was an answer to prayer. All we knew was she had to be pretty special to capture Luke's attention.

It took a little more than one month for my dad to have his catheter removed and be transferred to rehab, but this again was an amazing miracle, as the doctors had claimed that his digestive system, urinary tract, and bowels would probably never function again. Once a month, Larry and I traveled from Yakima to the Portland/Vancouver area for me to stay with my dad while Larry went to visit with his aging mother. While I stayed with Dad over the weekend, my mother took the opportunity to go home and catch up on things there.

This was an amazing bonding time for the two of us. My dad and I have always had a special understanding between one another. I felt as if I could share some of my issues of deliverance and confide in him that I was praying for his complete freedom as well. Journal entry October 14, 2018:

"I am so thankful & grateful, Father, for all the details & creative powers You are demonstrating in my dad's life-YES! It is frustrating that he can't get up & do what

he wants to, in fact, depend on others for his day-to-day needs & activities & can't even say what he wants. He is so determined, yet through all of these sufferings, You are doing amazing healing in his body & more importantly, in his soul & spirit. I know he will come out of this all completely transformed for Your glory & for the benefit of him & all of our family."

Even though my dad couldn't speak, I could see the understanding in his eyes. Often, he'd tear up, and I could sense a softness coming over him. He met regularly with a speech therapist, who worked mostly on swallowing skills, and also with an occupational and physical therapist. By Thanksgiving, he was able to have his feeding tube removed from his stomach and move into an assisted living facility. Since he and my mom had a two-level home with upstairs bathrooms, there was no way for my dad to return home without a miracle. With practice, my dad was eventually able to get in and out of the car so my mom could transport him to appointments and other places. One of his favorite trips was to visit her mother, his dear mother-in-law, who spent the entire time holding my dad's hand.

Since prepared meals were included with the rent, my mom decided to pay the extra fee and become a resident herself at the facility, but this still meant traveling back and forth to care for their home. She appreciated my monthly trips to give her a break.

Each time I came, I accompanied my dad to all his therapy sessions. Eventually, he was able to walk short distances with a brace on his right leg and a hemi-walker, as long as he was secured with a gait belt for balance. I occasionally took his guitar and secured it on his lap. As he was still paralyzed on the right side, I would strum the strings for him, and my dad was able to use his left hand to form and play chords. He couldn't talk, read, or write but could play guitar chords perfectly. He would always appreciate me reading scripture and singing with him. He got to the place where we could hum in harmony. At times, we would practice the harmonica together. It took a lot of determination and effort for him, but I believe he felt the satisfaction of his accomplishments.

In October 2019, my beautiful, dear, praying grandmother was called home to be with Jesus at age 103 years, 7 months, and 11 days. She was surrounded by my mom, dad, uncle, and aunt, who were singing her favorite hymns as she slipped into eternity. No fighting, no pain. Since Grandma had more friends than could be counted, it was decided to hold her memorial service the following March on her birthday weekend. That would give time to inform relatives and friends, and there would not be concern for travel on winter highways.

Lucas continued to keep in close contact with Heather, and shortly after my grandmother's death, we heard that he took a detour from his trucking schedule to visit with her dad. Larry and I were quite curious about the event. Shortly after, our suspicions were confirmed. Lucas had asked for and been granted Heather's hand in marriage.

Lucas left his trucking job in December to come with Heather to the Pacific Northwest and share a week's vacation with Larry and me on beautiful Mt. Hood. He had designed a special engagement ring for Heather, which he presented to her at that time. The more we got to know her, the more we loved her. We ended the vacation by celebrating my parents' 60th wedding anniversary. It was held in a big community hall at their assisted living facility. It was a great time for Lucas to introduce Heather to the family.

Even though the day wore my dad out, he and my mom so enjoyed all the friends and family who came to congratulate and honor them. My dad couldn't talk, but his eyes said it all. His pride was replaced with love. Haughtiness was replaced with compassion and kindness. Instead of looks of judgment, there was a softness in his eyes, fully accepting of others. My dad had always been so independent and private. Now, everything was exposed for everyone to see. It was necessary for him to depend on others. The man who never wanted to be pampered was housed in assisted living; however, there wasn't an ounce of anger or frustration on his face. He appeared to be bathed in peace. We continued to pray for a miracle, but I knew God had already completed the biggest miracle of all in my dad.

"Just as a father has compassion on his children,
So the Lord has compassion
on those who fear Him.
He Himself knows our form;
He is mindful that we are but dust."
Psalms 103:13-14

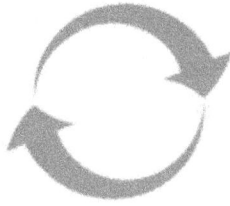

Chapter 25

TIME TO BUILD

As the 2020 New Year kicked off, I felt a stirring inside of me. I could see that things were rapidly moving to the left with my job. The LGBQT movement was growing, the Woke culture was just getting off the ground, and our outreach office from the clinic was supporting the entire agenda. I knew the time would come when taking a stand for righteousness could cost me my job. I didn't know how or when, but I was prepared.

In January, we moved Larry's mom from her independent home in Oregon to a senior living facility in Puget Sound. She needed to be closer to family as she was demonstrating increased signs of dementia, and Larry's brother was her financial adviser. The new home had 24-hour staff who could assist her with daily living.

Larry and I realized we, too, were getting older. We lived in a 55+ senior park, but rent continued increasing. I decided to do some research on our property in Central Oregon. I wondered if, after retirement, maybe it would be a smart idea to build a duplex there, and when our missionary kids were in the area, they'd have a place to stay. It was February 3, 2020. I looked up our property on the county map and found it was zoned R-5. I looked up the details online and discovered that they fell under the category of group homes. Immediately, I heard,

"It's not for you. It's a recovery home for women." Wow, that was totally unexpected! Out of curiosity, I looked up group homes online, and the first picture that popped up was the most beautiful home I had ever seen. It was three stories, with a deck on the front and back with spacious living areas on each floor. My mind started to rationalize and figure out how to cut corners to save money. Once again, I immediately heard, "Aren't they worth it?" These precious women could watch the sunrise come up from the east on the back deck. They could watch the sunset over the west mountains from the front deck. It would be a place filled with love and healing, a cleft in the rock.

When Larry and I first moved to Yakima with no jobs, we threw around the idea of starting a home of safe refuge for kids, and Larry had come up with the name "A Cleft in the Rock." Now, God was bringing it all back to memory, including the verse He had planted in my spirit down in South America. Proverbs 24:27: **"Prepare your work outside and make it ready for yourself in the field, afterwards, then build your house."**

I knew this idea didn't come from me. In every direction I searched, it seemed that pieces of the puzzle were falling into my lap. I shared the vision with Larry, and he also became excited. He could take care of maintenance and cooking. We needed confirmation. On February 16, we arrived early to church. Larry and I were in the car discussing the ministry and prayed for God to make His plan clear. That day, our pastor felt he needed to change his planned sermon. He instead preached, "God fights when I move." I cried through the whole message. It was clear. That week, we filed our name with the Oregon State Business Registry. It seemed as if we were in a self-propelled warp zone. With the help of some friends, we filed our articles of incorporation.

March 7, 2020, was Grandma's celebration of life. The place was filled with lots of precious pictures, videos, and shared stories. All our family was there, including our newest member, Heather. It was a beautiful day to remember and honor a woman who had impacted thousands not only in America but around the world. After the memorial, Larry and I shared our vision for "A Cleft in the Rock" with my parents. My mom was full of questions but excited. My dad was visibly touched as he broke out into tears. I knew they'd be faithful prayer partners for the ministry.

Then COVID hit. In a moment, everything was closed down. You know the story. Churches were told not to meet, flights were canceled, and businesses went under. Both my parents' and Larry's mom's facilities were locked to visitors and family. The public was gripped with fear. The vision was just as strong in my heart, but I knew, just like the children of Israel, I needed to wait for the cloud, but it seemed to have stopped for now. We didn't want to move ahead in the flesh.

I knew that if we were to move to Oregon, we would need to sell our house. Now was the time to get that ready. We dug into some renovation projects. Larry seemed to be on board. Much of the time, the house was disorderly, dusty, and difficult to maneuver in, but thankfully, Larry remained patient. He had never been one to deal well with change, but I was seeing a new side of him. I was witnessing, for the first time, patience and self-control being demonstrated in his life. When I was tired, Larry picked up the slack without criticizing or complaining.

Lucas and Heather decided to get married on her parents' property in the Appalachian Mountains of Virginia. They carefully planned a three-day "Shindig" with camping, BBQs, games, dancing, and a tree-planting ceremony to conclude with their wedding vows. It was scheduled for July 10-12, 2020, right in the heart of COVID. The crowd was smaller, but the celebration couldn't have been any more beautiful or festive. Heather has the most gracious and hospitable parents, and their property is situated in the heart of a southern oasis. Lucas had a pastor friend from Arizona who made the trip to officiate the ceremony. He and his wife have been mentors to Lucas and Heather ever since.

In August, I was invited to attend Samuel's wedding. He had resigned from his internship at my clinic and had plans for his honeymoon to tour the national parks with his new bride. What a great way to escape the COVID madness! It was a beautiful wedding, and as I observed their happy faces, I realized God's faithfulness in this young man's life and His desire for restoration and wholeness in all our lives.

Later that month, Larry and I were invited to attend another wedding of one of our original boys from Sunshine Acres, Mark. He and his bride were married in Idaho, near Boise. He was the oldest of the first three brothers to enter our home in Saguaro Hill. They were all there for the celebration. Mark had found a beautiful lady with a very loving and supportive family. We all realized their future ahead would be much different from that of his beginning. We had a great time of reunion, reminiscing, and counting all of our blessings over the years.

Several years back, Larry and I heard about a historic hotel in Spokane, the Davenport. It sounded enchanting, so we planned to celebrate our 40th wedding anniversary there. Our children had received word of our wishes and decided to pay for our elegant room, joining us for a weekend celebration in Spokane. They rented a separate house and invited other close family members to come to surprise us with a memorable time together for our anniversary. December 6, 2020, marked 40 years for Larry and I. We were presented with a beautiful carved wooden sign introducing "A Cleft in the Rock."

It was a wonderful gesture from our children, agreeing with us in faith for our upcoming home—a treasure indeed! It was a very special day of recounting God's care for our family. Larry and I felt very grateful, blessed, loved, and honored.

Later, after returning to our room, Larry and I continued to reminisce over past years and discuss the events of our lives together. We were in agreement that if we knew back at the beginning what we knew now, we would still have done it all over again. The love we now shared after 40 years of marriage was stronger than ever before. We learned to show love and respect for one another from the heart. We both discovered that by releasing our mates to be the people God created them to be and supporting them in the journey, we could experience fulfillment and be more united than ever. We knew it was only by the grace of God and our individual choices to obey and forgive.

That week after returning to work, I was asked to take a COVID test. I knew our clinic was receiving thousands of dollars throughout this "crisis." We, as employees, were given large bonus checks for being "essential workers." I felt a nauseated feeling in the pit of my stomach as if I was receiving blood money. Our doors were closed to the public. We were conducting all our business over the phone. I wasn't sick, had no symptoms, and felt no reason to be tested. I declined and was asked in response to go home for 14 days to quarantine. Our CEO had major differences with my Christian and political convictions. To make a long story short, my quarantine was extended to 41 days, and I was eventually fired in February 2021 over the whole incident. Once again, God, in His goodness, had prepared me ahead of time.

I wondered if this could be the time for the cloud to set out, but it didn't seem so. We continued working on our home remodeling projects while I began looking for work. In April, I was hired by a company providing housing for those who were in substance abuse treatment or who had finished the program and were in recovery. The agency agreed to hire me without the COVID vaccination and assured me it wouldn't be required in the future. So, it seemed I was receiving on

-the-job training for our women's home and being paid for it at the same time. God is good!

"Now faith is the assurance
of things hoped for,
The conviction of things not seen."
Hebrews 11:1

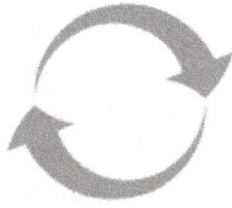

Chapter 26

ANOTHER TIME AROUND?

So, I dove in head-first, anxious to learn the ropes in my new job. I was responsible for managing an apartment complex, all the while enforcing the clean and sober model. I found myself stepping up to the plate in a new way. It was necessary for me to evict tenants and go to court for non-compliance. I could sense this role was indeed preparing me for what might lie ahead for "A Cleft in the Rock."

I had wondered throughout the years if my personal story and struggles could help other women. Who knows? Perhaps the life lessons I learned might even be an encouragement to the women who would move into the women's home. That summer, I consciously began writing my thoughts down on paper.

It appeared as if things were going smoother in our private life. Other than normal aches and pains from aging, Larry and I were feeling well. My husband was more comfortable getting out of the house, joining me for church events, giving his ideas and input, and praying with me about the recovery home. I felt like trust was being rebuilt in our relationship. I was grateful, but was this all too good to be true?

One morning, I remember lying in bed, halfway asleep. I was thanking God for His faithfulness and many answers to prayer over the years. I recalled all of His amazing attributes:

His goodness, kindness, and patience. I thanked Him for being caring and humble. Wait. I was just about to apologize when I heard God say, "I appreciate that you understand that about Me." Huh? I knew that Jesus was humble. In fact, He said if we want to be great in God's kingdom, we need to be the servant of all. But God the Father? Was He also humble? When Jesus was asked by His disciples to show them the Father, Jesus answered that if they had seen Him, they'd seen the Father. Jesus was demonstrating His Father's character of humility. Wow! What a new insight.

We have an enemy who wants to keep us as far away from humility as possible. He's called the "father of lies" and he's very good at tempting us to be selfish and prideful, to defend ourselves and want our own way. We think we're better or smarter than others. At times, we, as God's children, take the bait, stray off the path, and get disoriented. When we sin either knowingly or ignorantly, it breaks our fellowship with God and robs our peace and joy. God is more willing than us to restore our relationship. Jesus is called the Good Shepherd because He leaves all the rest of the sheep behind to seek us out. He never gives up. When we become aware of our error and are willing to repent and to be teachable, we can get back on track. Thank God, it's not three strikes and you're out! It says in 1 John 1:9, **"If we confess our sins, He is faithful and righteous to forgive us our sins and to cleanse us from all unrighteousness."** God is all about relationships. It warms His heart.

Our life has a ripple effect. What we do affects others in ways we may never know. We might have good intentions, but in the end, we do it all wrong. As hard as we may try, we can't control our surroundings, situations, or others. Thankfully, we have an amazing God who sees and knows all. He's aware of our pitfalls ahead of time, yet doesn't control His creation. He offers us advice for the path of abundant life but allows us free choice.

The God of all the universe chose to come to Earth in the form of the Son, limit Himself to experience human frailties, walk in our shoes, and participate firsthand in what human life is like. He thought it through well before stepping out of eternity into our fallen existence. To Him, it was worth the pain and suffering to feel our hurts.

The only payment for sin is death. We've all gone our own way, rejected God, and done life according to our plans. Jesus took that punishment of death for me, for you. He died on the cross and, even through the anguish, cried out to His Father, "Forgive them. They don't know what they're doing!" He was buried and lay there for three days. The good news is that He's not still in that grave. He victoriously arose, spent time with his depressed followers for 40 days, and after encouraging them, returned to His Father to make a fantastic home of celebration for us all. Now, He's watching and praying for us. Nothing goes unnoticed.

In Greek, the word for salvation is SOZO. It not only means to save from sins but also to heal and deliver. God plans for His children to experience the fullness of His salvation right now. It's a tragedy to live a miserable life on Earth, just hanging on by our fingernails until the day He snatches us out of our wretched existence and transitions us to Heaven. No, Jesus suffered and died for us to have our sins forgiven, and He endured the agony so we could live fully free here and now.

Life is hard. Life isn't fair. You may say, "I don't believe in God. I've never seen any evidence of His care in my life." That's what our enemy, the devil, wants you to believe. He's a liar, a killer, and a destroyer. His goal is to snuff you out for good. God says in Jeremiah 29:11-14, **"'For I know the plans that I have for you,' declares the Lord, 'plans for prosperity and not for disaster, to give you a future and a hope. Then you will call upon Me and come and pray to Me, and I will listen to you. And you will seek**

Me and find Me when you search for Me with all your heart. I will let Myself be found by you,' declares the Lord...'" He doesn't promise to take us out of the storm, but He promises to be with us in the middle of it. Believe it or not, He can truly give amazing peace when everything around is swirling out of control. Proverbs 15:15: **"All the days of the afflicted are bad, but a cheerful heart has a continual feast."** He's a miracle worker!

It seemed that Larry and I had finally worked out a plan for our financial disasters. He'd been paying his own bills for a few years at this point. I had no reason to believe there was any problem. In June 2021, Larry asked to talk to me about a situation. He informed me that we would be receiving numerous phone calls and I shouldn't answer. Larry disclosed that he was over his head in debt and had contacted Debt Blue, a debt settlement company. He owed several thousand dollars in credit card debt and was no longer able to make the minimum payments. The settlement company had made arrangements, and, with their help, Larry would make his agreed-upon monthly payment to be able to pay off his balances in four years. This was all too familiar, and I understood.

Later, while thinking about this conversation, I was reminded of a similar conversation I had with God prior to moving to Arizona. I had felt betrayed and lied to and no longer trusted Larry; *"GOD! I thought I was finally starting to see light at the end of the tunnel! Now I feel like I am just going around the same circle again! I can't take this!"* I also clearly remembered God's kind response, *"If I ask you to go around the circle one more time, will you trust Me?"* *"Yes"* was my resolution. *"I will and I <u>do</u> trust You."*

The interesting thing is the magnitude of the incident described by Larry earlier in the day was SO much bigger than that of my previous recollection, yet I was fine. Back in 1999, I felt as if my world was crashing down around me. What had made the difference? Romans 2:1 warns, **"Therefore you have no excuse, every one of you who passes judgement, for in that which you judge another, you condemn yourself, for you who judge practice the same things."**

Could it be that I had blamed all the dysfunction on Larry while I was equally to blame? Or maybe I was just doing my best to keep all my ducks in a row and frustrated at the impossible task? Amazingly, somewhere between 1999 and today, through my act of trust, God gently lifted me off the merry-go-round of craziness and held me tight. During the past 22 years, He allowed me to let go of everything that wasn't of Him and just rest. What once overwhelmed and appeared insurmountable and impossible for me seemed of little significance now. I could relate to the psalmist David when he scribed Psalm 30:11-12: **"You have turned my mourning into dancing for me; You have untied my sackcloth and encircled me with joy, that my soul may sing praise to You and not be silent. Lord my God, I will give thanks to You forever."**

Instead of being frustrated, I actually was proud of Larry. Yes, he'd taken the initiative to be responsible for his actions and was putting no blame on me. He was humble and had made a plan to solve his dilemma. My husband included me in the process, not to put pressure on me but to ask for my support. As the Lord tarried, Larry agreed to work and pay toward his financial obligation until it was settled. If all went as planned, he'd be free from his debt at age 73, but as I had continued to believe, I now felt assured that this time, he would succeed.

Gratitude and peace filled my heart. After all these years, despite the difficult process, I was once again given the opportunity to rebuild my hope and trust in Larry as the head of our home.

No, thankfully, I'm confident that I'll never be going around that circle again.

"So, as those who have been chosen of God,
Holy and beloved, put on a heart of compassion,
Kindness, humility, gentleness, and patience;
Bearing with one another,
and forgiving each other,
Whoever has a complaint against anyone;
Just as the Lord forgave you,
So also should you."
Colossians 3:12-13

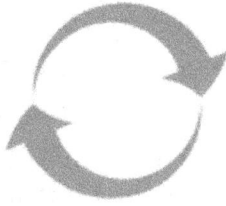

Chapter 27

DAYS TO CHERISH

I continued working into the fall, applying my experience and learning new skills on the job with Triumph Treatment. What I didn't anticipate was the pressure that was being increasingly placed on businesses. My new employer was now being told by the State of Washington to test all employees weekly for COVID if they'd not taken the vaccination. Once again, I was forced to make a choice; to bow or take a stand. I made it a matter of prayer, and in October, 6 months into my new job, I found myself again facing no employment.

However, God, in His ultimate wisdom, had creatively paved a brilliant path of provision for our family. The night before my last day of work at the treatment center, I received a phone call from my sister. My mom had just suffered a brain hemorrhage. She was in the hospital, and my dad was alone in the care center, unable to walk or talk. The doctors were brainstorming the plan of action, contemplating brain surgery. My husband and I jumped into the car and drove the four-hour drive to the hospital in Portland, Oregon, where my mom was conscious. The bleeding had stopped. The damage was minimal, but she would need help for her recovery.

My brother lived locally and was a big help, but his full-time job kept him busy. My sister also lived close by, but she was currently out of the country. My siblings asked if I would consider caring for my parents and offered a daily stipend to cover our expenses. Larry and I discussed and prayed about the options. It was clear that God had opened this door of opportunity. We were in agreement. I was amazed as my husband and I returned home for me to briefly pack my bags, preparing to leave Larry behind and return to be with my parents that weekend. The plan was to care for them both throughout the end of the year. I was beyond grateful for Larry's support. I now had the time and ability to focus my attention on doing what I could to help my parents.

So, my role and daily routine quickly changed to that of caregiver, counselor, and transporter for both of my parents. My dad continued his busy schedule of daily speech and PT but also began a new regimen of weekly Procrit shots to increase the hemoglobin in his blood. In September, a bone marrow test revealed that Dad wasn't producing white blood cells and platelets normally. The doctors didn't give him long to live without the shots. All our family came together and agreed in prayer for health and healing for both my parents.

My mom had Physical Therapy, Occupational Therapy, and Home Health come to see her regularly, but shortly after I came to stay, she suffered another headache and returned to the hospital, where she had several tests done. Through the MRI, the doctors confirmed my mom had an older hemorrhage several months prior that had healed. There also appeared to be new areas that were leaking. Their idea was that her vessels were becoming weak, and episodes of high blood pressure were causing the leakage. This impacted her vision, balance, and reasoning. The plan of action was to check her blood pressure often and keep the pressure lower by medication.

During those days together, I had numerous opportunities to pray, encourage, read scripture, participate in meals, and play games with my parents. I gave updates on my plans for "A Cleft in the Rock." As he'd done previously, my dad showed his approval by shedding tears of joy. Both he and my mom were supportive and excited about the vision God had placed in my heart. My mom quickly regained her strength and balance, and the plan to keep her blood pressure under control seemed to prevent further bleeding. By the end of the year, she was feeling better, and we were starting to get on one another's nerves.

Larry and I would arrange weekends to see each other monthly, including our 41st anniversary celebration in December. On one of those weekend rendezvous, I had time to think and pray as I drove towards home. I remember thanking God for the opportunity to care for my parents. I was in awe of all the ways Larry had changed in recent years and his willingness to let me stay with them these past few months without placing any guilt on me, with no complaint or attempt to control me. I recalled the prior years of ugliness, abuse, and a man who was seemingly selfish and unwilling to let me be myself. As I prayed and praised, I experienced a life-changing revelation.

God reminded me of the kind-hearted man who had driven to help me with my weekly Bible club many years back. I became aware of the pressure I had put on Larry to be the husband I wanted, rather than encouraging him to be the man he was created to be. Proverbs 12:4 admonishes, **"An excellent wife is the crown of her husband, but she who shames him is like rottenness in his bones."** In those first years, I forced Larry back into a corner. In trying to fight to retain his identity, he did all he knew to survive. I pushed him to become the angry man who resented me. Instead of showing excellence and love, I often shamed and belittled my husband.

As memories of Larry's cruel words and actions came to mind, I realized that now, instead of hurtful words, it was more common for him to give compliments. Rather than pressuring me to keep a tidy house, he was willing to jump in and help with daily chores, prepare meals, and be patient with my unfinished projects that are often left scattered around our home. I surely witnessed a true miracle of supernatural transformation. Once again, I was keenly aware that God is pleased by WHO we are rather than WHAT we do. That day, back in Chile, when I released my controlling hands from my husband, spiritual chains fell off us both so that we could be free. That weekend, after returning home, I asked for Larry's forgiveness. Thankfully, he was quick and gracious to forgive.

At the end of my three-month commitment, Larry joined our family as we celebrated my dad's 81st birthday together in their home on New Year's 2022. It was a day of rejoicing as we recounted God's faithfulness in all our lives. Afterward, I packed my bags to return home permanently to Yakima to join my husband and once again pick up where I left off in the search for employment.

I applied diligently and interviewed for numerous jobs for which I was well qualified but found no success. During this time, I prayed and researched online to gather more ideas for the women's home. During my search, I repeatedly came across information that seemed to highlight trafficked victims. Hmm... God had made it clear that the home was for women in recovery. Trafficked women surely needed a place to recover. This led me to ask God more about the matter and to clarify the commission. Again, I was excited to see God was leading the way, and if I kept following the breadcrumbs, I would find the treasure. It was also becoming clear to me, through all the COVID governmental regulations, that this was a home that God wanted to build without any fiscal red tape. I was definitely OK with that, but this meant praying and asking for God to stretch me in new areas of faith.

I continued to apply for work with no response until I was

phoned on March 1 by the director of a homeless camp and offered a job as a case manager. Camp Hope is a Christian homeless camp, where there's freedom to offer the hope of Jesus to hurting residents. I was delighted to join the team. I shared an office with a wonderful co-worker, who consequently specialized in working with human trafficking victims! So, once again, I had the opportunity for on-the-job training.

Despite my dad's weekly shots, his strength declined, and he was taken to the hospital emergency room routinely. It was necessary to give him blood transfusions to keep his blood levels in a safe range. He was experiencing severe pain that seemed to be in his bones, and we wondered if it was due to the shots. In June, he decided not to return to the ER, to no longer receive blood, and to stop his Procrit shots. Despite the pain, Dad was kind and amazingly patient. He continued speech and PT as long as he was able. Even though it was an effort, he tried his best to smile for caregivers and everyone who visited. On Father's Day, I was able to share a special time with my parents, sister, and aunt. It was one of the last days he would be able to eat on his own. I shared with my parents the update on "A Cleft in the Rock." Once again, my dad shed tears of affirmation and joy. On July 20, my dad left us to join His Lord and Savior, Jesus Christ. He was ready. He was an example to all of us who watched as he finished his race well.

On September 10, 2022, we had Dad's memorial service at my parents' church. My mom and all four of us children shared precious memories. The service can be seen online at http://vimeo.com/theneighborhoodchurch/doyal. We're not sure if he was watching, but we pray it was honoring for him.

"For this perishable must put on the
imperishable,
And this mortal must put on immortality.
But when this perishable will have put on the
imperishable,
And this mortal will have put on immortality,
Then will come about the saying that is written:
'Death is swallowed up in victory.'"
1 Corinthians 15:53-54

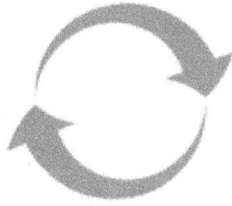

Chapter 28

More Than Imagined

I can't recall how long I've had the desire. I'm certain it's been decades of thinking about and praying for the opportunity. After making the move to Yakima, I connected with various individuals who've ministered in the local jails. I questioned some of them about the process for being approved to go in myself and visit with the inmates. The opportunity never transpired, but when the COVID mandates were ushered in, even the well-seasoned volunteers were unable to continue their routines or enter the facilities.

After completing a year of work at Camp Hope as a case manager, I was asked to move to an outreach position, which entailed working off-property. Soon after, Yakima County organized and started a resource group of providers to work with inmates targeted for discharge. The plan was to work on individual goals and facilitate a successful re-entry back into the community. In order for me to participate with the providers, the country initiated my background check and assisted in completing all needed documentation for me to enter the jail. I was excited to go in and participate with agencies on a weekly basis and even more delighted when I discovered I could schedule professional visits to meet with inmates privately. I began spending an entire day there once a week.

I would arrange visits with those who were a part of our resource group, but I could schedule from names on the jail roster of others I had met in the community and recognized throughout the years while working with the homeless and vulnerable population. It was also exciting to visit with people I had never met before. It didn't take long for me to see the various ways that God would direct the appointments. I would always look forward to my day at the jail to participate in conversations that uplifted and encouraged the individuals.

One day, a new lady, Lola, came to meet with me. I introduced myself and explained that I was there to offer resources and encouragement. I asked her what she had been interrupted from when the officer brought her to our visit. She reported that she had been reading a Bible that was left in her cell. I asked where she was reading, and she responded that she didn't know, but she had opened it up to the center. I asked if it might have been Psalms, and she said, "Maybe." I questioned if she knew who the author of Psalms was, and she said, "No." We began a dialogue about David's life as a shepherd boy, God's love and care for him, and how he became a famous king. Lola was mesmerized and full of questions. I, too, was amazed as God personally revealed Himself to her.

For a moment, I felt as if I could relate to the account of Philip in Acts 8, when he visited with the Ethiopian eunuch, explaining to him the book of Isaiah. It was the same Holy Spirit who was leading our conversation right there in the jail. I was an eyewitness that day of God's interest and care in the details of Lola's life. It was a divine appointment orchestrated by God Himself. I left in awe and wonder, anticipating the next visit.

Years prior, while wondering about God's direction for my life, I contemplated training with YWAM and asked Him the question, "Is this what You have planned for me?" I distinctly remember His answer: ***"You can't imagine what I have planned for you!"***

Back then, I was so naïve. I had lofty ideas and thought I knew what was best for me, my marriage, my family, and my ministry. I thought I had done a pretty good job in planning things out, and I was sure I would be able to help God with the details. I didn't have a clue of the valuable lessons that would lie ahead and what would transpire throughout my school of life. Had the plan been left to me, I would never have learned about the struggles of mental illness and the rewards of forgiveness. I had been taught as a child that God was my provider, but if I had not traveled down my own difficult road, I wouldn't have experienced the benefits of reaping and sowing and seeing firsthand the miracles of His provision for my family. God did and continues to truly accomplish the best for us all, so much more than I could ever have imagined!

God was gracious in allowing my husband to pay off his financial debt two years earlier than anticipated. Larry, in turn, expressed his thanks to me for my patience and support over the years. He described the way that God had confirmed to him my talent for budgeting. Larry was sincere when he told me he appreciated my help and asked me to finally take charge of our household financial matters going forward. At his request, I agreed. God is good.

Larry's freedom from debt at age 71 has enabled him to fully retire from employment and enjoy life. After announcing his retirement, we found ourselves singing together in worship service, "Bless the Lord, Oh my soul, and all that is within me, bless His holy Name." I held Larry's hand as I reflected back over the years. I was reminded of my life 15 years prior. Here in Yakima, I was finally able to trust and share my life with others. This is where I found accountability and support. The result of exposing our secrets to the light was deliverance from abusive patterns of relating to one another. I recounted numerous times when God had set me free from thought patterns and false beliefs. I recalled the years I experienced hopelessness and depression, 30 years prior, actually begging God to take my life. God had ministered hope during that time while I prayed for my husband. The chorus continued, "He has done great things, He has done great things, He has done great things, bless His holy Name!"

Even though I had presumed so much about God back then and did things my own way, He has always been so good and faithful to us both. All I can say is our marriage is a true testament to the faithfulness, grace, and mercy of our God. The horizon certainly looks different today than it did when we began...and no, I can't imagine what still lies ahead!

But as it is written,
"Eye hath not seen, nor ear heard,
Neither have entered into the heart of man,
The things which God hath prepared for them
that love him."
I Corinthians 2:9 KJV

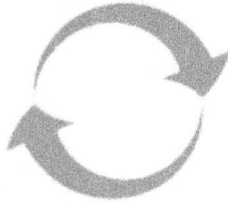

Chapter 29

WAITING ON THE WIND

For most of my life, when I set my mind to do something, not much can stop me. I can be very determined.

When God gave the vision for the women's home, it seemed that everything fell together so quickly, but after a year of silence, I was becoming a bit impatient. I knew that I didn't want to step ahead on my own. I had learned my lesson on presumption and making decisions by logic. I was also reminded of the story in Genesis 16, of the way that Abraham had messed things up by growing impatient with God. When he was told that he and his wife Sarah would have a son in his old age, he took matters into his own hands and bore his son, Ishmael, through Sarah's handmaiden. Boy, did that cause a load of trouble going forward!

When we set up our bylaws for "A Cleft in the Rock," our son, Lucas, and daughter-in-law, Heather, agreed to be founding members of the non-profit. This meant that we would meet yearly to go over the ministry details.

Heather shared a dream that she had with me. She saw a sailboat on a lake. The wind was pushing it along at a fast clip, but then the breeze stopped. The area was completely calm as the boat rocked gently on the crystal-clear water. Heather believed that this was the place where I was now. Instead of experiencing frustration, it was a time to be calm, pray, listen, and wait. Once again, when the wind filled the sails, and the boat took off, I had to be ready.

I was reading in 2 Samuel 7, describing David's excitement for building God a house, but God told him his son would be the one to build the temple instead. David then put all the preparations into motion and gave the commission to his son, Solomon. As I continued reading about the construction of the temple in 1 Kings 6, I learned that after taking the throne, Solomon took four years before he even began to build the temple and then seven more years to finish it. OK, I got the picture. I just needed to relax and take a deep breath!

I remember myself as that passionate 20-year-old who was rip-raring to go. I thought I was ready then, but I had so many things to learn. When I started out in marriage, I had so many thoughts, ideas, opinions, and false beliefs I needed to be set free from. Jesus said in John 10:27, **"My sheep hear My voice, and I know them, and they follow Me."** I knew a lot about God back then but still had set out in the wrong direction. Perhaps I had somehow created my own "Ishmael." What else do I need to learn? What remains in the darkness from which I need deliverance? How do I need to prepare? What important lessons does God still want to teach me?

I know God's priority is to have intimacy with me. He says in Jeremiah 9:23-24, **"Thus says the Lord, 'Let not a wise man boast of his wisdom, and let not the mighty man boast of his might, let not a rich man boast of his riches; but let him who boasts boast of this, that he understands and knows Me, that I am the Lord who exercises lovingkindness, justice and righteousness on the Earth; for I delight in these things,' declares the Lord."** I want my main focus to be knowing Him and to stay on course. I am determined to follow His lead.

Hebrews 11 is full of examples of heroes of the faith who

were asked to step out of their comfort zones and accomplish amazing feats for God. Many of them took on the challenge, never seeing the fruit of their labor before they died. That's what real faith is: believing without ever seeing.

When we purchased our vacation property in 1981, we thought it was for us, maybe for vacation or retirement. My parents bought the two acres bordering our property the following year. My dad made it a project to build a tree house and swing for the grandchildren. Both of our plots were improved by building outhouses for our personal use. Not much more was done to add value. After my dad's passing, we learned that my parents had written into their will and testament for their property in Central Oregon to go to Larry and me upon their death. Now that my dad was gone, my mom made the decision to pass the land on to Larry and me before her own death. We now have four acres available for the development of the women's home.

It seemed as if there were so many years that were wasted. I thought I needed to be mature and have all my credentials in place before I could be used of God. I expected things to be made right with others first and for reconciliation. The devil wants to keep us paralyzed and numb, to keep us in a state of slumber, to never step out in faith. That way, we're not a threat to the devil or an asset to anybody.

Originally, I thought we would apply for government grants to build the women's home, but through the process of waiting and praying, I now believe God may want to provide another way. Psalms 127 says, **"Unless the Lord builds the house, they labor in vain who build it."** He sees the completed plan. He owns it all. He's the ultimate provider. Who knows? This book may even be used by God to call someone to jump onboard the sailboat.

None of us are promised tomorrow. If there's anything I've learned over my lifetime, it's important to not miss a moment. I must make the most of every opportunity today. In the meantime, I'll continue working, building relationships, learning, and ministering to the residents of Camp Hope. I don't take for granted the blessing God has given us as a family. Both of our mothers currently need our support and encouragement in their later years. Larry and I are thankful for the opportunity to be with, love, and care for our parents for as long as they need us.

And I'll wait on the wind.

"Do not boast about tomorrow,
For you do not know what a day may bring forth."
Proverbs 27:1

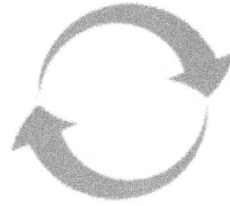

Chapter 30

The Path Ahead

Although uncomfortable, one constant is change. January 2024 ushered in an unexpected chain of events. My mother-in-law took a fall that rendered her unable to return to her assisted living apartment in Puget Sound. After a careful search, Larry and his brother decided to move her to an Alzheimer's home in Yakima, near Larry and me. We were now able to see her regularly and spend less time traveling to the Seattle area.

My mom has always been very active and health-conscious, so we were surprised to learn of her diagnosis of stage 4 cancer in autumn of the same year. Sometimes life throws unexpected roadblocks and detours along the way, and we don't arrive at our anticipated destination in our planned time frame, but Hebrews 6:10 promises, **"God is not unjust so as to forget your work and the love which you have shown toward His name, in having ministered and in still ministering to the saints."** He is faithful in leading us every step of the journey.

December 2024 marked 44 years of marriage for my husband and me. On our wedding day, how could I have ever imagined what lay ahead for us? At this point in life, maybe you're anticipating an announcement that Larry and I are both totally healed and now have a marriage made in heaven. Definitely NOT the truth ... sorry. I'm still the very stubborn and independent oldest child in the family, and Larry continues to struggle with quite a short fuse. We have loads of room to grow. The good news is that we've finally both submitted our wills to our Heavenly Father and are working really hard on submitting to one another.

I recall seasons in years past when I wallowed in self-pity, and all I wished for was to escape my misery. Now, instead of complaints and petitions, I'm full of praise and gratitude. Rather than placing unfair expectations on one another, Larry and I are learning to celebrate our differences and the unique talents and interests God has placed in our souls. I'm taking my calling seriously to be a vessel for showing God's love to my husband, and he, in turn, is being very creative in doing the little things to prove he really does love me. His words and actions are building a convincing case!

God doesn't promise any of us an easy life, but He gives us encouragement in John 16:33, **"These things I have spoken to you, so that in Me you may have peace. In the world you have tribulation, but take courage; I have overcome the world."**

After completing this manuscript, I read my story to Larry in person for the first time. He wasn't aware of most of my feelings or my personal memories until then. He didn't even remember many of my detailed recollections. We shed tears together as we reminisced about our shared events, good and bad, over the years, but there was no hurt, blame, or anger. Larry shared my hope that our story could be an instrument of healing for others. He asked to give his input on the foreword to show his support. We each expressed our love and thankfulness to one another and to our caring God, who made the miracle of our marriage possible.

Larry and I are taking Proverbs 18:21 to heart: **"Death and life are in the power of the tongue, and those who love it will eat its fruit."** We're doing our best to make it a habit to bless and pray for one another out loud daily. This has made a huge difference in how we see and believe in and for each other. One thing I'm sure of: Larry isn't the same person I married many years back. I'm totally honest in saying he's grown and matured into a kinder and more sensitive man. I hope he can report the same about me.

Prior to her move, while traveling the long road back home after visiting his mother, Larry asked to share with me a revelation God had recently shown him. I was delighted as he detailed the examples of God's intimate care by giving him the blueprint through the Bible for living a fulfilled life. Our eyes welled with tears as we thanked God together for wanting the best for us but giving us free will and allowing us to trust and follow His loving guidelines for abundant living. I assured my husband that he was the apple of God's eye and that I'm pretty sure he's God's favorite. After some quiet reflection, Larry began singing an old chorus:

"Oh, how He loves me and you. Oh, how He loves me and you. He gave His life. What more could He do? Oh, how He loves me. Oh, how he loves you. Oh, how He loves me and you!"

I joined in the duet as we sang together for several minutes, reveling in our Father's affirmation and presence. There's nothing more healing than the love of God.

I'm convinced that every single thing we've encountered in life has been for our good. God sees the beginning from the end and is every bit trustworthy. He truly can take what was meant for evil and turn it into good. His love is all-encompassing and never, ever ends. I'm honored and privileged, with God's help, to love my husband while sharing and growing with him into our golden years.

I thank God for reminding me years back about the testimony of the wife who had declared God's will over her husband. He honored her faith and set her husband free. I was tempted many times to give up in my time of deep pain. Instead, I accepted the challenge and tried it for myself. I chose to pray, trust, and declare God's will over my husband. Today, I can also testify to the power of agreeing with God.

Last 4th of July, we spent the day celebrating with our family late into the evening. Grandpa played games with the kids. They laughed and had a great time, and Larry didn't wear out or get frustrated even once. He told me later that he had not taken his medication that day, and I wondered if, some time in the future, he might not need it.

This scenario is becoming the norm rather than the exception. Larry is becoming more sensitive and attentive to the feelings of others. When he loses his temper, Larry is quick to ask forgiveness. Could God, after all these years, finally be healing my husband of his mental illness?

When our children were young, I prayed over their future spouses, for God to prepare, protect, and provide for them as they grew. Despite Lucas' vow to never marry, we've witnessed the seemingly impossible. We're thankful for the treasure of my beautiful daughter-in-law, Heather, who's an important part of our family. Lucas and Heather have made it a habit to practice quarterly getaways to celebrate their marriage relationship. This next summer will mark five years of matrimony for them. To add irony to the mix, they recently shared their own vision to facilitate getaways for other married pastors and missionaries around the globe. They made plans to leave this spring for various foreign continents to invest in the gift of marriage with some of these couples. I anticipate exciting new adventures on their horizon.

A benefit of social media is staying in contact with and continuing to be involved in the lives of our children from Sunshine Acres. One of our boys contacts us weekly for evening devotion time and to share advice and encouragement. These kids are all grown up now with families of their own. I'm visibly seeing the equity of investing in my marriage, our children, and extended families. We are witnessing the fruit of investing in the Kingdom of Heaven. I'm not worthy of God's goodness and faithfulness. I'm so humbled and thankful, and I am certain that these benefits will continue into the next generation.

The other night, I sat in the living room, commenting to Larry that we might be a rare family. Larry and I, along with our children and their spouses, have been through mission training and have served practical time overseas in mission work. I believe my childhood vision of being a missionary is truly being realized in more ways than I initially dreamed. As of today, I've had the privilege of traveling to and serving in 17 foreign countries and numerous Caribbean Islands, many of them together with Larry.

The COVID craziness has changed many things. Actually, I believe life will probably never return to the way it was before. I do have confidence, though, that somehow, one day soon, the foundation will be laid, and a beautiful house will be built for hurting women to be welcomed into a safe refuge to experience salvation, healing, and deliverance at "A Cleft in the Rock." God promises in 1 Thessalonians 5:24, **"Faithful is He who calls you, and He also will bring it to pass."**

I've learned to no longer presume on God, His timing, plans, or purposes. Even though I'm pressing on toward a vision and destination, I want to pay close attention, enjoy the journey, and take full advantage of every opportunity along the way. Every life is valuable and worthy of my stopping to make time to listen. If I'm patient and mindful to "stop and smell the roses." so to speak, I know God will continue to surprise me with special treasures to share with others.

I'm reminded of the message that drew me back to God those many years back. He told me the Bible was true, He was real, and that Jesus is coming back soon. I believe this more than ever, and the time is definitely closer now than when I was 19 years old. I'm intently preparing for, planning, and looking forward to His return. In the meantime, I'll keep my eyes out for the opportunities. I'm willing and available to share my life story with others, hoping that they might learn from my experiences and possibly avoid years of going around in endless circles like I did.

We all have different paths to travel. You may or may not be able to relate to my story, or maybe you've experienced things I can't begin to understand. Neglect, abandonment, rejection, and abuse can cripple and prevent an individual from being able or wanting to continue on. All I know is that forgiveness is a miracle.

Maybe you've never believed in Jesus as your personal Lord and Savior. That's the place to start. Our Father God sent His only begotten Son to come to Earth to be born of a woman. Jesus is fully God and fully man, but perfect and without sin. He said in John 14:6, **"I am the way, and the truth and the life; no one comes to the Father, but through Me."** Our sin separates us from God. The punishment for sin is death.

Jesus suffered and died on a cruel cross and was buried, but three days later, He rose again. He took the terrible punishment so that we can escape the power of sin and death, not only for eternity but for now. His sacrifice is the only provision we need to be saved. It's simple. Just believe that Jesus paid the full price. Accept His gift of forgiveness and confess with your mouth that He is not only THE Lord and Savior, but YOUR Lord and Savior. If you do that for yourself, you'll become a new creation, a child of God. He'll place His Holy Spirit inside of you, be your counselor and friend, and teach you His ways. He'll give you the desire and ability to forgive yourself and others. You'll see your path through new lenses.

One of my favorite life verses is Proverbs 4:18. I like to paraphrase it this way: **"The path of the righteous is like the breaking of the dawn that shines brighter and brighter until the light of full day."**

What is God trusting you for? Just as I was previously unaware of the daily opportunities, gifts, and talents that God had placed in my hands, He's given unique abilities to you to accomplish amazing feats for His Kingdom. Today is the day to step out in faith and make a difference. You don't need to wait until you are older or wiser. An impressive degree or a large social media following is not required. All God asks for is trust and obedience.

As of today, 2025 has fully kicked itself into gear. Time has wings. None of us are promised tomorrow. Many things are unknown about my future, but as long as I have breath, this I can promise: Larry and I are now traveling in the same direction, on the same path side by side, arms locked, determined, and united for one purpose. As long as we stay humble and united, we'll win. Through the blood of Jesus and His ongoing changing power in our lives, we won't be going around any more circles. We're racing toward the finish line as a team. Nothing will stop us. The farther we go, the lighter it gets!

I pray the same for you.

In the name of Jesus Christ, our Savior and Healer, be blessed!

"The Lord bless you, and keep you;
The Lord cause His face shine on you,
And be gracious to you;
The Lord lift up His countenance on you,
And give you peace."
Numbers 6:24-26

Dear Larry,
You're God's favorite.
He sure loves you.
So do I.

www.ingramcontent.com/pod-product-compliance
Lightning Source LLC
Chambersburg PA
CBHW070111030426
42335CB00016B/2111